Clinical Skills for OSCEs

D0314837

Clinical Skills for OSCEs

Neel L. Burton
BSc (Hons), MBBS, AKC

Akbar H. de' Medici
BSc (Hons), MBBS, PhD

Nicholas C. Stacey
BSc (Hons), MBBS, AKC

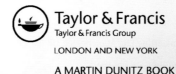
Taylor & Francis
Taylor & Francis Group

LONDON AND NEW YORK

A MARTIN DUNITZ BOOK

© 2003, 2005 BIOS, an imprint of the Taylor & Francis Group

First published in the United Kingdom in 2003 by BIOS, an imprint of the Taylor & Francis Group,
2 Park Square, Milton Park, Abingdon, Oxon OX14 4RN

Tel.:	+44 (0) 207 017 6000
Fax.:	+44 (0) 207 017 6699
E-mail:	info@dunitz.co.uk
Website:	http://www.tandf.co.uk

Reprinted 2005

A CIP record for this book is available from the British Library.

ISBN 1 85996 340 4

Distributed in North and South America by

Taylor & Francis
2000 NW Corporate Blvd
Boca Raton, FL 33431, USA

Within Continental USA
Tel: *800 272 7737; Fax:*   *800 374 3401*
Outside Continental USA
Tel: *561 994 0555; Fax:*   *561 361 6018*
E-mail: *orders@crcpress.com*

Distributed in the rest of the world by
Thomson Publishing Services
Cheriton House
North Way
Andover, Hampshire SP10 5BE, UK
Tel.:   +44 (0)1264 332424
E-mail: salesorder.tandf@thomsonpublishingservices.co.uk

Typeset by Servis Filmsetting Ltd, Manchester, UK

Printed by Biddles Ltd, Kings Lynn, UK

Life is short, the art long, opportunity fleeting, experiment treacherous, judgement difficult.

Hippocrates (c. 460–370 BC). Aphorisms, Aph. 1.

Contents

Psychiatry

ENT and ophthalmology

Paediatrics

Geriatrics

Dermatology

Obstetrics and gynaecology

Preface

Clinical skills exams, such as Objective Structured Clinical Examinations (OSCEs), are a daunting but essential component of medical undergraduate education.

To prepare for these exams, our generation of medical students had to pull together vast amounts of information from maladapted resources. This tedious and time-consuming process can now be avoided, as all this information has been compiled into this one, handy book.

Indeed, this book covers all the clinical skills that are likely to be tested during the clinical years of a medical course. Although it aims to be comprehensive and detailed, its primary purpose is to be easy to read and to the point. *Clinical Skills for OSCEs* does *not* attempt to teach its reader medicine or surgery, but rather gathers and organises a large amount of information and presents it in a structured and memorable fashion.

We hope you find *Clinical Skills for OSCEs* useful both for your revision and for the consolidation of skills learnt at the patient's bedside.

Neel L. Burton
Akbar H. de' Medici
Nicholas C. Stacey

London, August 2002

1. Take a blood pressure

Before starting

Introduce yourself to the patient.

Explain the procedure and ask for his consent to carry it out.

Inform him that he might feel some discomfort as the cuff is inflated, and that the blood pressure measurement may have to be repeated.

The procedure

- Position the patient's arm so that it is horizontal at the level of the mid-sternum.
- Place the vertical column so that it is at eye level.
- Locate the brachial artery at about 2 cm above the antecubital fossa.
- Select an appropriately sized cuff and apply it to the arm, ensuring that it fits securely.
- Inflate the cuff to 20–30 mmHg more than the estimated systolic blood pressure. You can estimate the systolic pressure by palpating the brachial artery pulse and inflating the cuff until you can no longer feel it.
- Place the stethoscope over the brachial artery pulse, ensuring that it does not touch the cuff.
- Reduce the pressure in the cuff at a rate of 2–3 mmHg per second.
  - The first consistent Korotkov sounds indicate the systolic blood pressure.
  - The muffling and disappearance of the Korotkov sounds indicate the diastolic blood pressure.
- Record the blood pressure as the systolic reading over the diastolic reading. Do not attempt to "round off" your readings.
- If the blood pressure is higher than 140/90, indicate that you might take a second reading after giving the patient a one minute rest.

! **If the patient has a history of postural hypotension, you must also record the standing blood pressure.**

After the procedure

Ensure that the patient is comfortable.

Tell the patient his blood pressure and explain its significance.

Thank the patient.

2. Perform a venepuncture

Specifications: The station consists of an anatomical arm and all the equipment that might be required. Assume that the anatomical arm is a patient and take blood from it.

Before starting

Introduce yourself to the patient.

Explain the procedure and ask for his consent to carry it out.

Ensure that he is comfortable.

The equipment

In a tray, gather:

- A pair of gloves.
- A tourniquet.
- Alcohol wipes.
- A 12G needle and a needle-holder.
- The bottles appropriate for the tests that you are sending for (these vary from hospital to hospital – learn them!).
- Cotton wool.

! Remember to ensure that you have a sharps bin close at hand.

The procedure

- Select a vein.
- Apply the tourniquet, and re-check the vein.
- Put on gloves.
- Clean the venepuncture site using the alcohol wipes.
- Attach the needle to the needle holder, and place a bottle on the needle holder.
- Tell the patient to expect a "sharp scratch".
- Retract the skin to stabilise the vein and insert the needle into the vein.
- Let the first bottle fill and then change bottles.
- Undo the tourniquet.
- Remove the needle from the vein and apply pressure on the puncture site.
- Dispose of the needle in the sharps bin.
- Remove gloves.

After the procedure

Ensure that the patient is comfortable.

Thank the patient.

Label the bottles (patient's name, date of birth, and hospital number).

Fill in the form (patient's name, date of birth, and hospital number, and the tests required).

3. Cannulate and set up a drip

This station is likely to require you either to cannulate an anatomical arm and to put up a drip, or simply to cannulate the anatomical arm. This chapter covers both scenarios.

Before starting

Introduce yourself to the patient.

Explain the procedure and ask for his consent to carry it out.

Gather equipment in a tray.

Cannulate only

The equipment

- A pair of gloves.
- A tourniquet.
- Alcohol swabs.
- An IV cannula of appropriate size (18G or bigger).
- A syringe containing saline flush.
- An adhesive plaster.
- A sharps box.

The procedure

- Find a suitable vein. Try to avoid the dorsum of the hand and the antecubital fossa.
- Apply the tourniquet to the arm and re-verify the vein.
- Put on the gloves.
- Clean the skin and let it dry.
- Remove the cannula from its packaging.
- Tell the patient to expect a "sharp scratch".
- Anchor the vein by stretching the skin and insert the cannula at an angle of about 30 degrees.
- Once flashback is seen, advance the entire cannula (needle and cannula) by 2 mm.
- Keep the needle fixed and advance the cannula into the vein.
- Remove the tourniquet.
- Press on the vein over the tip of the cannula, remove the needle, and cap the cannula.
- Immediately put the needle into the sharps box.
- Apply the adhesive plaster to fix the cannula.
- Flush the cannula.

After the procedure

Discard any rubbish.

Ensure that the patient is comfortable.

Thank the patient.

Cannulate and put up a drip

The equipment

- A pair of gloves.
- A tourniquet.
- Alcohol swabs.
- An IV cannula of appropriate size (18G or bigger).
- An adhesive plaster.
- A sharps box.
- An appropriate fluid bag.
- A giving set.

The procedure

- Check the fluid in the bag and the fluid prescription chart (if appropriate).
- Attach the giving set to the fluid bag and ensure that the giving set is run through.
- Find a suitable vein. Try to avoid the dorsum of the hand and the antecubital fossa.
- Apply the tourniquet to the arm and re-verify the vein.
- Put on the gloves.
- Clean the skin and let it dry.
- Remove the cannula from its packaging.
- Tell the patient to expect a "sharp scratch".
- Anchor the vein by stretching the skin and insert the cannula at an angle of about 30 degrees.
- Once flashback is seen, advance the entire cannula (needle and cannula) by 2 mm.
- Keep the needle fixed and advance the cannula into the vein.
- Remove the tourniquet.
- Press on the vein over the tip of the cannula and remove the needle.
- Immediately put the needle into the sharps box.
- Attach the giving set.
- Apply the adhesive plaster to fix the cannula.
- Adjust the drip-rate (1 drop per second is equivalent to about 1 litre per 6 hours).

After the procedure

Ensure that the patient is comfortable.

Thank the patient.

Discard any rubbish.

Make a recording on the fluid chart (if appropriate).

4. Measure blood glucose

Introduce yourself to the patient.

Explain the procedure and ask for his consent to carry it out.

Establish when he last ate.

The equipment

In a tray, gather:

- A pair of gloves.
- An alcohol wipe.
- A glucose monitor.
- Test-strips.
- A spring-loaded pricker.
- A lancet.
- Cotton wool.

The procedure

- Ask the patient to wash and dry his hands, or use an alcohol wipe to clean the finger that you are going to prick.
- Massage the finger from its base to its tip to increase its perfusion.
- Turn on the glucose monitor and ensure that it is calibrated.
- Check that the test-strips have not expired.
- Insert a test-strip into the glucose monitor.
- Load the lancet into the pricker and prick the side of the finger.

! It is less painful to prick the side rather than the tip of a finger because there are comparatively fewer nerve endings there.

- Squeeze the finger to obtain a droplet of blood. If no or insufficient blood is obtained, prick the finger again.
- Place the droplet of blood on the test-strip, so as to cover the sensor entirely.
- Give the patient some cotton wool to stop any bleeding.
- Record reading. Units are millimoles per litre.

After the procedure

Tell the patient their blood glucose and explain its significance and any further action that needs to be taken.

Ask the patient if he has any questions or concerns.

Thank the patient.

Interpretation of results	
Capillary blood glucose	**(mmol/l)**
Normal	
fasting	<5.6
non-fasting	<7.8
Impaired fasting glucose	
fasting glucose	≥5.6 and ≤ 6.0
Diabetes mellitus	
fasting glucose	>6.0
non-fasting	>11.0

! All abnormal results must be confirmed by a laboratory measurement.

5. Test a urine sample

Before starting

Introduce yourself to the patient.

Take a very brief history from him.

Explain that you are going to test his urine and explain why.

Ensure that the urine specimen is fresh and that it has been appropriately collected.

The equipment

- Urine dipstick and urine dipstick bottle.
- A pair of gloves.
- A pen and paper (or the patient's notes).

The procedure

- Put on the gloves.
- Observe the colour and appearance of the urine.
- Stir the urine bottle to ensure that the urine is mixed.
- Check the expiry date of the urine dipsticks.
- Briefly immerse a urine dipstick into the urine specimen.
- Tap off any excess urine from the dipstick.
- Hold the strip horizontally.
- Read each colour pad at the designated time printed on the dipstick bottle colour chart.
- Report and record the results.
- Discard the used urine dipstick and the gloves.
- Wash your hands.

After testing the urine

Explain the results to the patient.

Thank the patient.

6. Scrub up for theatre

Before handwashing

State that you would change into theatre uniform.

Put on clogs or plastic overshoes.

Don a theatre cap, tucking all your hair beneath it.

Remove all items of jewellery, including your watch.

Enter the scrubbing room.

Put on a face mask. Ensure that it covers both your nose and mouth.

Open a sterile gown pack *without touching the gown*.

Lay out a pair of sterile gloves *without touching the gloves*.

Handwashing

▷ Open a brush packet.

▷ Open the taps.

! From here on, keep your hands above your elbows at all times.

The social wash

▷ Wash your hands with soap, lathering up your arms to 2 cm above the elbows.

The second wash

▷ Use the nail pick from the brush packet to clean under your fingernails.

▷ Dispense soap onto the sponge side of the brush and use the sponge to scrub from the fingertips to 2 cm above the elbows (30 seconds per arm).

! Dispense soap using your elbow or a foot pedal, not your hands.

▷ To rinse, start from your hands and move down to your elbows.

The third wash

▷ Using the brush side of the brush, scrub your fingernails (30 seconds per arm).

▷ Using the sponge side of the brush, scrub:

 ▷ Each finger and interdigital space in turn (30 seconds per arm).

 ▷ The palm and back of your hands (30 seconds per arm).

 ▷ Your forearm, moving up circumferentially to 2 cm above the elbows (30 seconds per arm).

! **Remember to keep the brush well soaped at all times.**

▷ To rinse, start from your hands and move down to your elbows

▷ Turn the taps off with your elbows.

After handwashing

Use the towels in the gown pack to dry your arms from the fingertips down.

Pick up the gown from the inside, ensuring that it does not touch anything.

Put your arms through the sleeves, but do not put your hands out of the cuffs.

Put on the gloves. Do not touch the outside of the gloves. (Practise this – it's not easy!)

Ask an assistant to tie up the gown.

! **After scrubbing up, keep your hands in front of your chest and do not touch any non-sterile areas, including your mask and hat.**

7. Catheterise a male patient

Specifications: A male anatomical model in lieu of a patient.

Before starting

Introduce yourself to the patient.

Explain the procedure and ask for his consent to carry it out.

Position him.

Gather the equipment onto a clean trolley.

The equipment

- A catheterisation pack.
- Antiseptic solution.
- Sterile gloves.
- 2% lignocaine gel.
- A 16 french Foley catheter.
- A catheter bag.
- A 10 ml saline-filled syringe.
- Adhesive tape.

The procedure

- Open the catheter pack aseptically, and pour antiseptic solution into the receiver.
- Wash and dry your hands.
- Put on sterile gloves.
- Drape the patient.
- Place a collecting vessel in the patient's *entre-jambes*.
- Hold the penis using a sterile swab.
- Retract the foreskin and clean the area around the urethral meatus.
- Insert the lignocaine gel into the urethra and hold the urethral meatus closed.
- Indicate that the anaesthetic needs about 5 minutes to work.
- Hold the penis so that it is vertical.
- Holding the catheter by its sleeve, gently and progressively insert it into the urethra.
- Inject 5 ml of saline to inflate the balloon, continually ensuring that this does not cause the patient any pain.
- Attach the catheter bag.
- Gently retract the catheter until a resistance is felt.
- Reposition the foreskin.
- Tape the catheter to the thigh.

After the procedure

Ensure that the patient is comfortable.

Thank the patient.

Discard any rubbish.

Record the volume of urine in the catheter bag.

8. Catheterise a female patient

Specifications: A female anatomical model in lieu of a patient.

Before starting

Introduce yourself to the patient.

Explain the procedure and ask for her consent to carry it out.

Position her.

Gather the equipment onto a clean trolley.

The equipment

- Two pairs of gloves.
- A catheterisation pack.
- Antiseptic solution.
- A 16 french Foley catheter.
- Lubricant jelly.
- A 10 ml saline-filled syringe.
- A catheter bag.
- Adhesive tape.

The procedure

- Open the catheter pack aseptically and pour antiseptic solution into the receiver.
- Wash and dry your hands.
- Put on both pairs of gloves.
- Drape the patient.
- Place a collecting vessel in the patient's *entre-jambes*.
- Use your non-dominant hand to separate the labia minora.
- Clean the area around the urethral meatus.
- Remove your outer gloves.
- Lubricate the tip of the catheter.
- Holding the catheter by its sleeve, gently and progressively insert it into the urethra.
- Inject 5 ml of saline to inflate the balloon, continually ensuring that this does not cause the patient any pain.
- Attach the catheter bag.
- Gently retract the catheter until a resistance is felt.
- Tape the catheter to the thigh.

After the procedure

Ensure that the patient is comfortable.

Thank the patient.

Discard any rubbish.

Record the volume of urine in the catheter bag.

9. Interpret a chest X-ray

A systematic approach to interpreting X-rays not only impresses the examiner, but also minimises yours chances of missing any abnormalities. Before saying anything, it is an excellent idea to spend one minute looking at the X-ray and organising your thoughts.

1. The X-ray

Name and age of the patient.

Date of X-ray.

PA or AP?

Erect or supine?

Rotation.

Penetration.

! **If penetration is normal, the upper half of the thoracic spine should be discernible.**

> ### Erect or supine?
>
> A radiograph can be confirmed as having been taken erect if the gastric air bubble lies under the left hemidiaphragm.
>
> AP films are almost invariably taken supine, and this has major implications for interpretation. A supine film differs from an erect film in that:
>
> - There is an enlarged heart size.
> - The diaphragm is higher, resulting in an apparent decrease in lung volume.
> - Pleural fluid levels lie vertically, resulting in an opacification of the lung field.
> - Any prominence of upper zone vessels does not suggest left heart failure.

2. Interventions

Make a note of any chest drains, ECG pads, etc., that may be visible on the X-ray.

3. The skeleton

Examine the ribs, the shoulder girdles and the spine.

4. The soft tissues

Examine the breasts, the chest wall and the soft tissues of the neck. Look for any distortion, and for any opacities and translucencies.

5. The lungs and hila

The lungs: Check the lung volumes, then carefully examine the lung fields, for any abnormal opacity or radiolucency.

The hila: Examine the hila, the densities created by the pulmonary arteries and the superior pulmonary veins of either lung for any abnormal opacities. Check their positions: the left hilum should be 1 cm higher than its right counterpart.

6. The pleura

Systematically check *all* lung margins, looking for pleural opacity, pleural displacement and loss of clarity of the pleural edge (the silhouette sign).

7. The mediastinum and heart

First look for any mediastinal shift. Then calculate the cardiothoracic ratio by dividing the maximal diameter of the heart by the maximal diameter of the chest. In a PA film this should be equivalent to 0.5 or less. Examine the trachea and right and left main bronchi. Then examine the aortic arch, the pulmonary artery and the heart. Are there any abnormal opacities (masses) or radiolucencies (pneumomediastinum)?

Most common conditions likely to come up in an *Interpret a chest X-ray* OSCE:

- Pneumonia.
- Pleural effusion.
- Emphysema.
- Pneumothorax.

- Lung cancer.
- Tuberculosis.
- Heart failure.
- Chronic obstructive pulmonary disease.

! Learn their signs.

10. Interview a patient with chest pain

Before starting

Introduce yourself to the patient.

Explain that you are going to ask him some questions to uncover the nature of his chest pain, and ask for his consent to do this.

Ensure that he is comfortable; if not, make sure that he is.

The history

- Name, age and occupation.

Presenting complaint and history of presenting complaint

- Ask about the nature of the chest pain. Use open questions.
- For any pain, determine its:
  - Nature.
  - Site.
  - Onset.
  - Duration.
  - Radiation.
  - Aggravating and alleviating factors (exercise, cold air, large meals, alcohol, movement etc.).
  - Associated symptoms and signs. Ask specifically about nausea and vomiting, shortness of breath, haemoptysis, cough and palpitations.
- Ask about any previous episodes of chest pain.

Past medical history

- Current, past and childhood illnesses. In particular, ask about coronary heart disease, cardiovascular accidents, hyperlipidaemia, hypertension, diabetes, deep vein thromboses, smoking, and alcohol consumption.
- Surgery.
- Recent visits to the doctor.

Drug history

- Prescribed medication. Ask specifically about the combined oral contraceptive pill.
- Over-the-counter drugs.
- Illicit drugs.
- Allergies.

Family history

◐ Parents, siblings and children. Ask specifically about heart disease.

Social history

◐ Foreign travel.

◐ Employment, past and present.

◐ Housing.

◐ Hobbies.

After taking the history

Ask the patient if there is anything that he might add that you have forgotten to ask. This is an excellent question to ask in clinical practice, and an even better one to ask in exams.

Thank the patient.

Summarise your findings and offer a differential diagnosis.

Say that you would like to examine the patient and order some investigations, for example, ECG and chest X-ray to confirm your diagnosis.

! **If you cannot differentiate angina from oesophagitis, advise a therapeutic trial of an antacid or a nitrate and/or record an ECG.**

Most common conditions likely to come up in an *Interview a patient with chest pain* OSCE:
◐ Angina.
◐ Gastro-oesophageal reflux disease.
◐ Chest infection.
◐ Pulmonary embolus.
◐ Musculoskeletal complaint.

11. Examine the cardiovascular system, including peripheral pulses

Before starting

Introduce yourself to the patient.

Explain the examination and ask for his consent to carry it out.

Position him at 45 degrees, and ask him to remove his top(s).

Ensure that he is comfortable.

The examination

General inspection

○ From the end of the couch, observe the patient's general appearance (age, state of health, nutritional status and any other obvious signs). Is the patient breathless or cyanosed?

○ Inspect the precordium for the presence of any abnormal pulsation and the chest for any scars. A median sternotomy might have been performed for coronary artery bypass grafting, for valve surgery, or for the repair of a congenital defect. Don't miss a pacemaker if it is there!

Inspection and examination of the hands

○ Take both hands noting:

  ○ Temperature.

  ○ Colour.

  ○ The presence of clubbing (endocarditis, cyanotic congential heart disease).

  ○ The presence of splinter haemorrhages (subacute infective endocarditis).

  ○ The presence of any nail signs (leukonychia – hypoalbuminaemia, koilonychia – iron deficiency).

○ Determine the rate, rhythm, and character of the radial pulse. Take the pulse in both arms (coarctation of the aorta).

○ Indicate that you might like to take a blood pressure measurement (see Chapter 1, *Take a blood pressure*).

Inspection and examination of the head and neck

○ Inspect the sclera for signs of anaemia.

○ Inspect the mouth for signs of central cyanosis.

○ Assess the jugular venous pressure and the jugular venous pulse form: having asked the patient to turn his head *slightly* to one side, look at the internal jugular vein medial to the clavicular head of sternocleidomastoid. Assuming that the patient is at 45 degrees, the vertical height of the JVP from the sternal notch should not be greater than 3 cm.

○ Locate the carotid pulse and assess its character.

! **Never palpate both carotid pulses simultaneously.**

Palpation of the heart

! **Ask the patient if he has any chest pain.**

○ Determine the location and character of the apex beat. It is normally located at the mid-clavicular line, at the level of the fifth intercostal space. A "tapping" apex beat indicates mitral stenosis; a "heaving" apex beat indicates left-ventricular hypertrophy.

○ Place your hand over the cardiac apex and on either side of the sternum and feel for any heaves and thrills.

Auscultation of the heart

○ Listen for heart sounds, additional sounds, murmurs and pericardial rub. Using the stethoscope's diaphragm, listen in:

  ○ The *aortic area*
    Right second costal intercostal space near the sternum.

  ○ The *pulmonary area*
    Left second costal intercostal space near the sternum.

  ○ The *tricuspid area*
    Left third, fourth, and fifth intercostal spaces near the sternum.

  ○ The *mitral area*
    Left fifth intercostal space, in the mid-clavicular line.

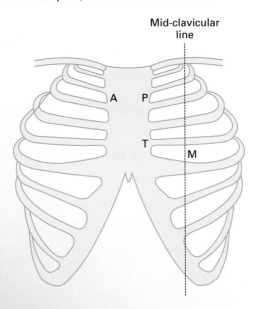

Figure 1. Auscultation points

In addition:

- Ask the patient to bend forward and to hold his breath in expiration. Using the stethoscope's diaphragm, listen at the left sternal edge in the fourth intercostal space for the mid-diastolic murmur of aortic regurgitation.
- Ask the patient to turn onto his left side and to hold his breath in expiration. Using the stethoscope's *bell*, listen in the mitral area for the mid-diastolic murmur of mitral stenosis.
- Listen over the carotid arteries for any bruits.

Common murmurs	
Aortic stenosis	Slow-rising pulse, heaving cardiac apex, mid-systolic murmur best heard in aortic area and radiating to carotids and cardiac apex.
Mitral regurgitation	Displaced, thrusting cardiac apex, pan-systolic murmur best heard in mitral area and radiating to axilla.
Aortic regurgitation	Collapsing pulse, thrusting cardiac apex, diastolic murmur best heard at left sternal edge.
Mitral valve prolapse	Mid-systolic click, late-systolic murmur best heard in mitral area.

Chest examination

- Percuss and auscultate the chest, especially at the bases of the lungs. Heart failure can cause pulmonary oedema and pleural effusions.

Abdominal examination

- Palpate the abdomen to exclude ascites and/or an enlarged liver.
- Check for the presence of an aortic aneurysm.
- Palpate the kidneys and listen for any renal artery bruits.

Ankle oedema

- Test for the dependent or "pitting" oedema of cardiac failure.

Peripheral pulses

- Feel the temperature of the feet and then palpate the:
  - Femoral pulses.
  - Popliteal pulses.
  - Posterior tibial pulses.
  - Dorsalis pedis pulses.

After the examination

Offer to test the urine and examine the retina by fundoscopy.

Cover the patient up.

Thank the patient.

Summarise your findings and offer a differential diagnosis.

Most common conditions likely to come up in an *Examine the cardiovascular system* OSCE:

- ◯ Murmurs. (See *Common murmurs* box).
- ◯ Heart failure.
- ◯ Median sternotomy scar.
- ◯ Pacemaker.

12. Examine the peripheral vascular system

In an OSCE, you might be asked to examine only the arterial or venous systems. You must, therefore, learn the signs that are relevant to either system.

Before starting

Introduce yourself to the patient.

Explain the examination and ask for his consent to carry it out.

Expose his legs, including his feet.

The examination

Inspection

▶ Skin changes: atrophy, pallor, shininess, pigmentation, loss of body hair.

▶ Scars.

▶ Signs of gangrene: black skin, nail infection, amputated toes.

▶ Venous and arterial ulcers. Remember to look in the interdigital spaces.

▶ Oedema.

▶ Varicose veins (ask the patient to stand up).

! **Do not make the common mistake of asking the patient to stand up before having examined for varicose veins.**

Palpation and special tests

▶ Skin temperature. Compare both legs.

▶ Capillary refill. Compress a nail bed for 5 seconds and let go. It should take less than 2 seconds for the nail bed to return to its normal colour.

▶ Peripheral pulses:

　▶ Femoral pulse at the inguinal ligament.

　▶ Popliteal pulse in the popliteal space (flex the knee).

　▶ Posterior tibial pulse behind the medial malleolus.

　▶ Dorsalis pedis pulse over the dorsum of the foot, just lateral to the extensor tendon of the great toe.

▶ Buerger's test:

　▶ Lift both of the patient's legs to 45 degrees and note the change in skin colour.

　▶ Ask the patient to dangle his legs over the edge of the couch. If the arterial supply is normal, the original skin colour should return in less than 10 seconds.

- Oedema. Firm non-pitting oedema is a sign of chronic venous insufficiency.
- Varicose veins. Tenderness on palpation suggests thrombophlebitis.
- Trendelenburg's test:
  - Elevate leg at 90 degrees to drain the veins.
  - Apply a tourniquet around the upper thigh.
  - Ask the patient to stand up. The veins should gradually fill up in 30–35 seconds.
  - Release the tourniquet. Sudden additional filling of the veins indicates sapheno-femoral incompetence.

Auscultation

- Femoral arteries.
- Abdominal aorta.

After the examination

Thank the patient.

Summarise your findings and offer a differential diagnosis.

Most common conditions likely to come up in an *Examine the peripheral vascular system* OSCE:

- Chronic arterial insufficiency.
- Chronic venous insufficiency, varicose veins, and varicose eczema and ulceration.

13. Record an ECG/EKG

Before starting

Introduce yourself to the patient.

Explain the procedure to him, specifying that it is not painful, and ask him for his consent to carry it out.

Position him so that he is lying on a couch.

Ask him to expose his upper body and his ankles.

The equipment

- A 12-lead ECG machine.
- Electrode sticky pads.

The procedure

- Attach the electrode sticky pads as per the leads.
- Attach the limb leads, one on each limb. The longest leads attach to the legs, above the ankles, and the mid-length leads attach to the upper arms.
- Place the chest leads (the shortest leads) such that:
  - V1 is in the fourth intercostal space at the right sternal margin.
  - V2 is in the fourth intercostal space at the left sternal margin.
  - V3 is midway between V2 and V4.
  - V4 is in the fifth intercostal space in the left mid-clavicular line.
  - V5 is at the same horizontal level as V4, but in the anterior axillary line.
  - V6 is at the same horizontal level as V4, but in the mid-axillary line.
- Turn the ECG machine on and press on "Analyse ECG" or a similar button.

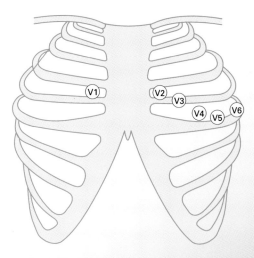

Figure 2. Lead placement

After recording the ECG

Check calibration and paper speed.

Analyse the ECG for any life-threatening abnormalities.

Remove the leads.

Discard the electrode sticky pads.

Ensure that the patient is comfortable.

Thank the patient.

14. Interview a patient with breathlessness

Introduce yourself to the patient.

Explain that you are going to ask him some questions to uncover the nature of his breathlessness, and ask for his consent to do this.

Ensure that he is comfortable; if not, make sure that he is.

The history

- Name, age and occupation.

Presenting complaint

- Ask about the nature of the breathlessness. Use open questions.

History of presenting complaint

Ask about:

- Onset, duration and variability of breathlessness.
- Provoking and relieving factors.
- Associated symptoms (wheeze, cough, sputum, fever, anorexia, loss of weight, haemoptysis, pain, faintness).
- Exercise tolerance.
- Sleep disturbance – can he lie flat?
- Smoking.

Past medical history

- Current, past and childhood illnesses, including asthma, atopy and tuberculosis.
- Surgery.
- Recent visits to the doctor.

Drug history

- Prescribed medication (especially NSAIDs and β-blockers).
- Over-the-counter drugs.
- Illicit drugs.
- Allergies.

Family history

○ Parents, siblings and children. Focus especially on respiratory diseases such as asthma, cystic fibrosis and emphysema (α1-antitrypsin deficiency).

Social history

○ Employment, past and present.

○ Housing.

○ Travel.

○ Alcohol consumption.

○ Hobbies (especially budgerigars and pigeons!).

After taking the history

Ask the patient if there is anything that he might add that you have forgotten to ask.

Thank the patient.

Summarise your findings and offer a differential diagnosis.

Say you would like to examine the patient and carry out some investigations to confirm your diagnosis.

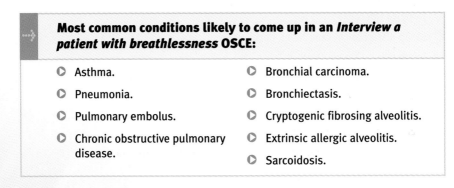

Most common conditions likely to come up in an *Interview a patient with breathlessness* OSCE:

○ Asthma.

○ Pneumonia.

○ Pulmonary embolus.

○ Chronic obstructive pulmonary disease.

○ Bronchial carcinoma.

○ Bronchiectasis.

○ Cryptogenic fibrosing alveolitis.

○ Extrinsic allergic alveolitis.

○ Sarcoidosis.

15. Examine the respiratory system

Introduce yourself to the patient.

Explain the examination and ask for his consent to carry it out.

Position him at 45 degrees, and ask him to remove his top(s).

Ensure that he is comfortable.

The examination

General inspection

○ From the end of the couch, observe the patient's general appearance (age, state of health, nutritional status and any other obvious signs). In particular, is he breathless or cyanosed? Does he have to sit up to breathe? Is his breathing audible? Is he coughing?

○ Note the rate, depth and regularity of the patient's breathing.

Note:

○ Any deformities of the chest (barrel chest, *pectus excavatum*, *pectus carinatum*) and spine.

○ Any asymmetry of chest expansion.

○ The use of accessory muscles of respiration.

○ Any operative scars.

Inspection and examination of the hands

○ Take both hands and assess them for colour and temperature.

○ Look for clubbing.

○ Determine the rate, rhythm, and character of the radial pulse. Is it the bounding pulse of carbon dioxide retention?

○ Test for asterixis, the flapping tremor of carbon dioxide retention.

The principal causes of clubbing	
Respiratory causes	Carcinoma Fibrosing alveolitis Chronic suppurative lung disease
Cardiac causes	Infective endocarditis Cyanotic heart disease
Hepatic causes	Cirrhosis
Gastrointestinal causes	Ulcerative colitis Crohn's disease Coeliac disease
Familial	

Inspection and examination of the head and neck

- Inspect the sclera for signs of anaemia.
- Inspect the mouth for signs of central cyanosis.
- Assess the jugular venous pressure and the jugular venous pulse form (cor pulmonale – right-sided heart failure).
- Palpate the cervical, supraclavicular, infraclavicular and axillary lymph nodes.

Palpation of the chest

Ask the patient if he has any chest pain.

- Palpate for tracheal deviation by placing the index and middle fingers of one hand on either side of the trachea in the suprasternal notch. Alternatively, place the index and annular fingers of one hand on either clavicular head and use your middle finger (called the *vulgaris* in Latin) to palpate the trachea.
- Palpate for the position of the cardiac apex.

Note: Carry out all subsequent steps on the front of the chest and, once this is done, repeat them on the back of the chest.

- Palpate for equal chest expansion, comparing one side to the other. Reduced unilateral chest expansion might be caused by pneumonia, pleural effusion, pneumothorax, and lung collapse. If there is a measuring tape, measure the chest expansion.
- Test for tactile fremitus by placing the flat of the hands on the chest and asking the patient to say, "ninety-nine".

Percussion of the chest

 Percuss the chest. Start at the apex of one lung, and compare one side to the other. Do not forget to percuss over the clavicles and on the sides of the chest. For any one area, is the resonance increased (emphysema, pneumothorax) or decreased (consolidation, fibrosis, fluid)?

Auscultation of the chest

 Ask the patient to take deep breaths through the mouth, and using the diaphragm of the stethoscope, auscultate the chest. Start at the apex of one lung, and compare one side to the other. Are the breath sounds vesicular or bronchial? Are there any added sounds?

 Test for vocal resonance by asking the patient to say, "ninety nine". If you have already tested for tactile fremitus, it is not necessary to test for vocal resonance.

After the examination

Ask to see the sputum pot.

Ask to measure the PEFR. (See Chapter 16, *Instruct on the use of a PEFR meter*).

Cover the patient up.

Thank the patient.

Summarise your findings and offer a differential diagnosis.

> **Most common conditions likely to come up in an *Examine the respiratory system* OSCE:**
>
> Chronic obstructive pulmonary disease.
>
> Pulmonary fibrosis.
>
> Lobectomy.

16. Instruct on the use of a PEFR meter

! **Also see *Explaining skills*, Chapter 85.**

Before starting

Introduce yourself to the patient.

Check his understanding of asthma.

Explain the importance of using a PEFR meter and the importance of using it correctly.

Explain that the PEFR meter is to be used first thing in the morning and at any time he has symptoms of asthma.

The skill

Ask the patient to (and demonstrate):

▶ Attach a clean mouthpiece to the meter.

▶ Slide the marker to the bottom of the numbered scale.

▶ Stand up or sit up straight.

▶ Take as deep a breath as possible and hold it.

▶ Insert the mouthpiece into his mouth, sealing his lips around the mouth piece.

▶ Exhale as hard as possible into the meter.

▶ Read and record the meter reading.

▶ Repeat the procedure three to six times, keeping only the highest score.

▶ Check this result against previous readings.

▶ Check the patient's understanding by asking him to carry out the procedure.

▶ Ask the patient if he has any questions or concerns.

17. Instruct on the use of an inhaler

! Also see *Explaining skills*, Chapter 85.

Before starting

Introduce yourself to the patient.

Check his understanding of asthma.

Explain that an inhaler device delivers aerosolised bronchodilator medication for inhalation and that, if used correctly, it provides fast and efficient relief from bronchospasm. Furthermore, it is relatively free of systemic side-effects.

Suggest reasons for the inhaler to be used.

The skill

Ask the patient to (and demonstrate):

- Vigorously shake the inhaler.
- Remove the cap from the mouthpiece.
- Hold the inhaler between index finger and thumb.
- Place the inhaler about 3–5 cm in front of his mouth.
- Breathe out completely.
- Breathe in deeply, and simultaneously activate the inhaler.
- Close his mouth and hold his breath for 10 seconds.
- Repeat the procedure after 1–5 minutes if relief is insufficient.
- Check the patient's understanding by asking him to carry out the procedure.

! If the patient has difficulty co-ordinating breathing in and inhaler activation, he may benefit from the added use of a spacer.

- Ask the patient if he has any questions or concerns.

18. Take a history of abdominal pain

Before starting

Introduce yourself to the patient.

Explain that you are going to ask him some questions to uncover the cause of his abdominal pain, and ask for his consent to do this.

Ensure that he is comfortable.

! **Ensure that the patient is *nil by mouth*. Acute abdomen is a surgical complaint and the patient must therefore be kept *nil by mouth* until the need for surgery has been excluded.**

The history

○ Name, age and occupation.

Presenting complaint and history of presenting complaint

○ Ask about the nature of the abdominal pain. Use open questions.

○ For any pain, try to determine:

  ○ Nature.

  ○ Site.

  ○ Onset.

  ○ Duration.

  ○ Radiation.

  ○ Aggravating and alleviating factors.

  ○ Associated symptoms and signs.

Ask about:

  ○ Fever.

  ○ Loss of weight.

  ○ Nausea and vomiting.

  ○ Anorexia.

  ○ Diarrhoea.

  ○ Constipation.

  ○ Melaena.

  ○ Steatorrhoea.

  ○ Indigestion.

  ○ Jaundice.

  ○ Genitourinary symptoms: frequency, dysuria, haematuria.

  ○ Last menstrual period.

Past medical history

- Previous episodes of abdominal pain.
- Current, past and childhood illnesses.
- Surgery.
- Recent visits to the doctor.

Drug history

- Prescribed medication.
- Over-the-counter drugs.
- Illicit drugs.
- Allergies.

Family history

- Parents, siblings and children. Ask specifically about colon cancer.

Social history

- Alcohol consumption.
- Smoking.
- Travel.
- Employment, past and present.
- Housing.

After taking the history

Ask the patient if there is anything that he might add that you have forgotten to ask.

Ask the patient if he has any questions or concerns.

Thank the patient.

State that you would carry out a full abdominal examination and order some key investigations such as urinalysis, serum analysis and an abdominal X-ray, as appropriate.

Summarise your findings and offer a differential diagnosis.

Most common conditions likely to come up in a *Take a history of abdominal pain* OSCE:

- Appendicitis.
- Gastro-oesophageal reflux disease.
- Peptic ulceration.
- Biliary colic.
- Acute cholecystitis.
- Ureteric colic.
- Acute pancreatitis.
- Diverticulitis.
- Colon cancer.

! Remember that basal pneumonia, diabetic ketoacidosis and an inferior myocardial infarct can also present as abdominal pain.

19. Take a urological history

Before starting

Introduce yourself to the patient.

Explain that you are going to ask him some questions to uncover the nature of his urological complaint, and ask for his consent to do this.

Ensure that he is comfortable.

The history

- Name, age and occupation.

Presenting complaint and history of presenting complaint

- Ask about main presenting complaint. Use open questions.
- Determine time course of events and the severity of the problem.
- Ask specifically about:
  - Pain. For any pain, ask about site, radiation, onset, duration, intensity, character, relieving and aggravating factors, and associated factors.
  - Fever.
  - Frequency.
  - Urgency.
  - Dysuria.
  - Haematuria.
  - Nocturia.
  - Hesitancy and terminal dribbling.
  - Incontinence.
  - Urethral discharge.
  - Sexual contacts.

Past medical history

- Past urological problems.
- Current, past and childhood illnesses.
- Surgery.
- Recent visits to the doctor.

Drug history

- Prescribed medication.
- Over-the-counter drugs.
- Illicit drugs.
- Allergies.

Family history

- Parents, siblings and children. In particular, has anyone in the family had a similar problem?

Social history

- Employment.
- Housing and home-help.
- Travel.
- Alcohol consumption.
- Smoking.

After taking the history

Ask the patient if there is anything he might add that you have forgotten to ask about.

Thank the patient.

If asked, summarise your findings and offer a differential diagnosis.

Most common conditions likely to come up in a *Take a urological history* OSCE:

- Urinary tract infection.
- Urinary incontinence.
- Prostatism.

20. Examine the abdomen

Before examining the patient

Introduce yourself to the patient.

Ask the patient for permission to examine his abdomen.

Say to the examiner that you would normally expose the patient from nipples to knees, but that in the OSCE you are going to limit yourself to exposing the patient to the groins.

Position the patient lying flat on the couch, with his arms at his side and his head supported by a pillow.

Ensure that the patient is comfortable.

The examination

General inspection

- From the end of the couch, observe the patient's general appearance (age, state of health, nutritional status and any other obvious signs).

- Inspect the abdomen for its contours and any obvious distension, localised masses, scars, skin changes. Ask the patient to lift his head to tense the abdominal muscles.

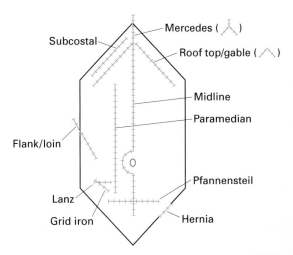

Figure 3. Abdominal scars

Inspection and examination of the hands

▶ Take both hands, looking for:

  ▶ Clubbing.

  ▶ Palmar erythema (liver disease).

  ▶ Duputyren's contracture (cirrhosis).

  ▶ Nail signs (leukonychia – hypoalbuminaemia, koilonychia – iron deficiency).

▶ Look for a liver flap (liver failure) by asking the patient to put out his hands and cock his wrists up.

Inspection and examination of the head, neck and upper body

▶ Inspect the sclera for signs of jaundice or anaemia.

▶ Inspect the mouth, looking for ulcers (Crohn's disease), angular stomatitis (nutritional deficiency), atrophic glossitis (iron deficiency, vitamin B12 deficiency, folate deficiency), furring of the tongue (loss of appetite) and the state of the dentition.

▶ Examine the neck for lymphadenopathy.

▶ Examine the upper body for gynaecomastia (cirrhosis) and spider naevia (chronic liver disease).

Palpation of the abdomen

! **Ask the patient if he has any abdominal pain and fix upon his face as you palpate his abdomen.**

▶ *Light palpation* – Begin by examining the segment furthest from any pain or discomfort and systematically palpate the four quadrants and the umbilical area. Look for tenderness, guarding and any masses.

▶ *Deep palpation* – For greater precision. Describe and localise any masses.

Palpation of the organs

▶ *Liver* – Ask the patient to breathe in and out and, starting in the right lower quadrant, feel for the liver edge using the flat of your hand. The liver edge, if felt, can be described in terms of regularity, nodularity and tenderness.

▶ *Gallbladder* – Palpate for tenderness over the gallbladder region, i.e. the tip of the ninth rib.

▶ *Spleen* – Palpate for the spleen as for the liver, again starting in the right lower quadrant.

▶ *Kidneys* – Position the patient close to the edge of the bed and ballot each kidney using the technique of deep bimanual palpation.

▶ *Aorta* – Palpate the descending aorta between the thumb and the index of one hand at a point midway between the xiphisternum and the umbilicus.

Percussion

- ▶ Percuss the liver area, also remembering to detect its upper border (usually found in the fourth intercostal space).
- ▶ Percuss the suprapubic area for dullness (bladder distension).
- ▶ If the abdomen is distended, test for shifting dullness (ascites).

Auscultation

- ▶ Auscultate in the mid-abdomen for abdominal sounds. Listen for 30 seconds before concluding that they are hyperactive, hypoactive or absent.
- ▶ Listen over the abdominal aorta for aortic bruits suggesting arteriosclerosis or an aneurysm.
- ▶ Listen for renal artery bruits, 2.5 cm above and lateral to the umbilicus – a bruit suggests renal artery stenosis.

! **The following are not usually performed in an *Examine the abdomen* OSCE, but they should be mentioned at this stage.**

Examination of the groins and genitals

(see Chapter 21, *Examine the male genitalia*)

Rectal examination

After the examination

Ask to test the urine.

Cover the patient up.

Thank the patient.

Summarise your findings and offer a differential diagnosis.

Most common conditions likely to come up in an *Examine the abdomen* OSCE:	
▶ Chronic liver disease.	▶ Renal transplant.
▶ Polycystic kidney.	▶ Scar(s).

21. Examine the male genitalia

Specifications: You may be asked to examine the male genitalia on a real patient or, more likely, on a pelvic mannequin.

Before starting

Introduce yourself to the patient.

Explain the examination and ask for his consent to carry it out.

Ask him to lie on the couch and expose his groin area.

Ensure that he is comfortable.

! **Ensure the patient's dignity at all times.**

The examination

General inspection

◉ From the end of the couch observe the patient's general appearance. The patient's age can give you an indication of the most likely pathology.

◉ In particular, note the distribution of facial, axillary and pubic hair.

◉ Look for gynaecomastia.

Inspection and examination of the male genitalia

◉ Warm your hands.

◉ Ensure that the patient is not in pain.

PENIS

◉ Inspect the penis for lesions and ulcers.

◉ Retract the foreskin and examine the glans penis and the external urethral meatus. Is there a discharge? Can a discharge be expressed?

  ◉ If there is a discharge, indicate that you would send it for microscopy and culture.

SCROTUM

◉ Inspect the scrotum. Are the testicles present? Is their lie normal? If a testicle is absent, is it retracted or undescended? If you find a scar, the absent testicle may have been surgically removed.

◉ Keep an eye on the patient's face and palpate:

  ◉ The testis.

  ◉ The epididymis.

  ◉ The vas deferens.

○ If you locate a mass, try to get above it. If you cannot it is likely to be a hernia. Test for a cough impulse.

○ Next, transilluminate the mass using a pen torch. Is it a cyst or a solid mass? If it is a cyst, is it a hydrocoele or an epididymal cyst? If it is a solid mass, is it tender? Is it testicular or epididymal?

○ If you suspect a varicocoele, a collection of varicosities in the pampiniform venous plexus, examine the patient in the standing position and test for a cough impulse. Note that varicocoeles are invariably left-sided.

Examination of the lymphatics

○ Palpate the inguinal nodes, in the inguinal crease. Only the penis and scrotum drain to the inguinal nodes, the testicles draining to the para-aortic lymph nodes.

After the examination

Cover the patient up.

Thank the patient.

Summarise your findings and offer a differential diagnosis.

Most common conditions likely to come up in an *Examine the male genitalia* OSCE:

○ Hydrocoele.

○ Epididymal cyst.

○ Varicocoele.

○ Direct inguinal hernia.

○ Penile ulcer(s).

22. Perform a rectal examination

Specifications: A plastic model in lieu of a patient.

Before starting

Introduce yourself to the patient.

Explain the procedure to him, emphasising that it might be uncomfortable but that it should not be painful, and ask for his consent to carry it out.

Request a chaperone, if appropriate.

Ask the patient to remove his trousers and underpants.

Ask him to lie on his left side, to bring his buttocks to the side of the couch, and to bring his knees up to his chest.

The examination

- Put on a pair of gloves.
- Gently separate the buttocks and inspect the anus and surrounding skin. In particular, look out for skin tags, excoriations, ulcers, fissures, prolapsed haemorrhoids, and mucosal prolapse.
- Lubricate the index finger of your right hand.
- Position the finger over the anus, as if pointing to the genitalia.
- Gently insert the finger into the anus, through the anal canal, and into the rectum.
- Test the anal tone by asking the patient to squeeze your finger.
- Rotate the finger so as to palpate the entire circumference of the anal canal and rectum. Feel for any masses, ulcers or induration.
  - In males pay specific attention to the size, surface and consistency of the prostate.
  - In females, the cervix can usually be palpated.
- Feel for the consistency of any faeces.
- Remove the finger and examine the glove. In particular look at the colour of the stool, and for any mucus or blood.
- Remove and dispose of the gloves.

After the examination

Clean off any lubricant or faeces on the anus or anal margin.

Give the patient time to put his clothes back on.

Address any questions or concerns that he might have.

Present your findings to the examiner, and offer a differential diagnosis.

23. Take a history of headaches

Before starting

Introduce yourself to the patient.

Explain that you are going to ask him some questions to uncover the nature of his headaches, and ask for his consent to do this.

Ensure that he is comfortable.

The history

▶ Name and age.

Presenting complaint and history of presenting complaint

First use open questions to get the patient's story.

Then ask specifically about:

▶ **S**ite.

▶ **O**rigin.

▶ **C**haracter.

▶ **R**adiation.

▶ **A**ssociated factors:

  ▶ Vomiting.

  ▶ Visual disturbances.

  ▶ Photophobia.

  ▶ GI disturbance.

  ▶ Fever.

  ▶ Rash.

  ▶ Tender temporal arteries.

  ▶ Neck pain.

  ▶ Altered level of consciousness.

  ▶ Neurological deficit.

▶ **T**iming

▶ **E**xacerbating and relieving factors (activity, caffeine, alcohol, dehydration, stress...)

▶ **S**everity (effect on patient's life).

SOCRATES (470–399 BC): *"I am not an Athenian or a Greek, but a citizen of the world."*

Drug history

○ Prescribed medication. Many drugs, including glyceryl trinitrate and calcium channel blockers, can cause headaches.

○ Over-the-counter drugs.

○ Illicit drugs.

○ Allergies.

Social history

○ Employment past and present.

○ Housing.

○ Mood. Depression is a common cause of headaches.

○ Smoking.

○ Alcohol consumption. Alcohol can cause headaches.

Past medical history

○ Current, past and childhood illnesses.

○ Surgery.

○ Recent visits to the doctor.

Family history

○ Parents, siblings and children.

After taking the history

Ask the patient if there is anything he might add that you have forgotten to ask about.

Ask the patient is he has any questions or concerns.

Thank the patient.

Summarise your findings and offer a differential diagnosis.

State that you would like to perform a physical examination and some investigations to confirm your diagnosis.

⤑ **Most common conditions likely to come up in a *Take a history of headaches* OSCE:**

○ Tension headaches.

○ Cluster headaches.

○ Migraines.

○ Cranial arteritis.

○ Cervical spondylosis.

○ Meningeal irritation.

○ Intracranial mass lesions, e.g., tumour.

○ Subarachnoid haemorrhage.

24. Take a history of a "funny turn"

Introduce yourself to the patient.

Explain that you are going to ask him some questions to uncover the cause of his collapse, and ask for his consent to do this.

Ensure that he is comfortable.

The history

- Name and age.

Presenting complaint and history of presenting complaint

First use open questions to get the patient's story.

Think about the commoner causes of a funny turn:

- Syncope
- Epilepsy
- Transient ischaemic attack
- Arrhythmia
- Postural hypotension (autonomic dysfunction, drugs)
- Carotid sinus syndrome
- Hypoglycaemia
- Vertebrobasiliar insufficiency

Ask about:

- If the patient remembers falling.
- The circumstances of the fall.
  - Had the patient just arisen from bed? (postural hypotension)
  - Did the patient suffer an intense emotion? (syncope)
  - Had the patient been coughing or straining? (syncope)
  - Had the patient been extending his neck? (vertebrobasilar insufficiency)
  - Did the patient have any palpitations? (arrhythmia)
- Any loss of consciousness and its duration.
- Prodromal symptoms such as aura, change in mood, strange feeling in the gut, sensation of déjà vu.
- Fitting, frothing at the mouth, tongue biting, incontinence.
- Headache or confusion upon recovery.
- Injuries sustained.
- Previous episodes.

Drug history

▶ Prescribed medication. Drugs such as phenothiazines, tricyclic antidepressants, and anti-hypertensives can cause postural hypotension. Insulin can cause hypoglycaemia.

▶ Over-the-counter drugs.

▶ Illicit drugs.

▶ Recent changes in medication.

Past medical history

▶ Current, past and childhood illnesses. Ask specifically about diabetes (autonomic neuropathy), epilepsy, heart problems, stroke, cervical spondylosis and arthritis.

▶ Surgery.

▶ Recent visits to the doctor.

Family history

▶ Parents, siblings, and children. Ask specifically about epilepsy and heart problems.

Social history

▶ Smoking.

▶ Alcohol consumption.

▶ Employment, past and present.

▶ Housing.

▶ Effect of fall(s) on patient's life.

After taking the history

Ask the patient if there is anything he might add that you have forgotten to ask about.

Ask the patient is he has any questions or concerns.

Thank the patient.

Summarise your findings and offer a differential diagnosis.

State that you would like to perform a physical examination and some investigations to confirm your diagnosis.

25. Examine the cranial nerves

Specifications: You will be asked to examine only a given number of cranial nerves, most likely cranial nerves V, VII and IX–XII.

Before starting

Introduce yourself to the patient.

Explain the examination and ask for his consent to carry it out.

Ensure that he is comfortable.

The examination

Inspection

The olfactory nerve

- Ask the patient if he has noticed a change in smelling or taste.

The optic nerve

(See *Examine vision and the eye*, Chapter 38, for more details.)

- Test visual acuity on a Snellen chart.
- Test near vision by asking the patient to read test types (or a page in a book).
- Indicate that you would use Ishihara plates to test colour vision.
- Test the visual fields by confrontation.
- Examine the eye by direct fundoscopy.

The oculomotor, trochlear and abducens nerves

(See *Examine vision and the eye*, Chapter 38, for more details.)

- Look for a ptosis (Horner's syndrome).
- Test the direct and consensual pupillary light reflexes.
- Test the accommodation reflex.
- Look for a visible squint.
- Ask the patient if he is seeing double.
- Perform a cover test.
- Test eye movements.
- Look for nystagmus.

The trigeminal nerve

SENSORY PART

- ▷ Test light touch in the three divisions of the trigeminal nerve. Test both sides.
- ▷ Indicate that you would test the corneal reflex.

MOTOR PART

- ▷ Test the muscles of mastication (the temporalis, masseter, and pterygoid muscles) by asking the patient to:
  - ▷ Clench his teeth. (Palpate temporalis and masseter muscles).
  - ▷ Open his mouth against resistance.
  - ▷ Close his mouth against resistance.
- ▷ Test the jaw jerk.

The facial nerve

- ▷ Look for facial asymmetry. The nasolabial folds and the angle of the mouth are especially indicative of facial asymmetry.
- ▷ Test the muscles of facial expression by asking the patient to:
  - ▷ Lift his eyebrows as far they will go.
  - ▷ Close his eyes as tightly as possible. (Try to open them).
  - ▷ Blow out his cheeks.
  - ▷ Purse his lips.
  - ▷ Show his teeth.

The acoustic nerve

(See *Examine hearing and the ear*, Chapter 37, for more details)

- ▷ Test hearing sensitivity in each ear.
- ▷ Indicate that you would perform the Rinne and Weber tests and examine the ears by auroscopy.

The glossopharyngeal nerve

- ▷ Indicate that you would test the gag reflex by touching the tonsillar fossae on both sides.

The vagus nerve

- ▷ Ask the patient to phonate (say "aaaaaah") and, aided by a pen torch, look for deviation of the uvula.

The hypoglossal nerve (cranial nerve XII)

- Aided by a pen torch, inspect the tongue for wasting and fasciculation.
- Ask the patient to stick out his tongue.

The accessory nerve (cranial nerve XI)

- Look for wasting of the sternocleidomastoid and trapezius muscles.
- Ask the patient to:
  - Shrug his shoulders against resistance.
  - Turn his head to either side against resistance.

After the examination

Thank the patient.

Summarise your findings and offer a differential diagnosis.

> **Most common conditions likely to come up in an *Examine the cranial nerves* OSCE:**
>
> - Third nerve palsy.
> - Bell's palsy.
> - Horner's syndrome.
> - Cavernous sinus lesion.
> - Cerebellopontine angle tumour.
> - Bulbar palsy.
> - Pseudo-bulbar palsy.
> - Brain-stem infarction.
> - Multiple sclerosis.
> - Motor neurone disease.
> - Myasthenia gravis.

26. Examine gait and co-ordination

Introduce yourself to the patient.

Explain the examination and ask for his consent to carry it out.

Examining gait

○ Ask the patient to stand up. Observe his posture and if he is steady on his feet.

○ Ask the patient to walk five or so paces and then to turn around and walk back. If he normally uses a stick or frame, he should do so. Observe the patient's arm swing and the individual components of the gait. Take special notice of how the patient turns around, as this requires good balance and co-ordination.

○ Heel-to-toe test: Ask the patient to walk heel-to-toe, as if on a tightrope.

○ Romberg's test: Ask the patient to stand unaided with his arms by his sides and with his eyes closed. If the patient sways and loses his balance, the test is positive (posterior column disease).

! **Be ready to catch the patient should he fall.**

Examining co-ordination

○ Ask the patient which is his dominant hand.

○ Look for a resting tremor in the hands.

○ Test tone in the arms.

○ Test for dysdiadochokinesis: Show the patient to clap and then to clap by alternating the palmar and dorsal surfaces of one hand. Ask him to do this as fast as he can. Repeat the test with his other hand.

○ Finger-to-nose test: Place your index finger at about two feet from the patient's face. Ask him to touch the tip of his nose and then the tip of your finger with his index finger. Ask him to do this as fast as he can. Repeat the test with his other hand. Intention tremor and past-pointing are signs of cerebellar disease.

○ Test fine finger movements: Ask the patient to oppose his thumb and each of his other fingers in turn. Ask him to do this as fast as he can. Repeat the test with his other hand.

○ Heel-to-shin test: Lie the patient on a couch. Ask him to run the heel of one leg down the shin of the other, and then to bring the heel back up to the knee and start again. Repeat the test with his other leg.

Ask the patient if he has any questions or concerns.

Thank the patient.

Summarise your findings and offer a differential diagnosis.

Most common conditions likely to come up in an *Examine the gait and co-ordination* OSCE:

- Parkinson's disease.
- Cerebellar ataxia.
- Sensory ataxia.
- Hemiplegia.
- Musculoskeletal disease.
- Senile gait.

27. Examine the sensory system of the upper limbs

Before starting

Introduce yourself to the patient.

Explain the examination and ask for his permission to carry it out.

Position him and ask him to expose his upper limbs.

The examination

To examine the sensory system, test light touch, pain, proprioception and vibration sense. Don't forget to inspect the arms before you start.

▶ **Light touch.** Ask the patient to close his eyes and apply a wisp of cotton or tissue to the sternum and then to each of the dermatomes of the arm. Compare both sides.

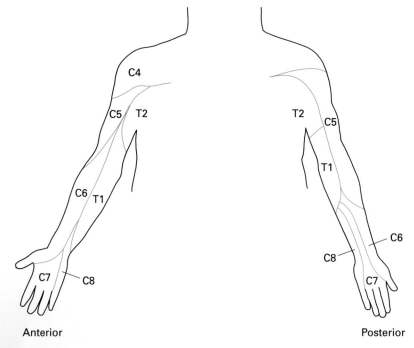

Anterior   Posterior

Figure 4. Dermatomes of the arm

▶ **Pain.** Ask the patient to close his eyes and apply a sharp object – ideally a neurological pin – to the sternum and then to each of the dermatomes of the arm. Compare both sides.

▶ **Proprioception.** Ask the patient to close his eyes. Hold one of his fingers by its sides and move it at the distal interphalangeal joint, asking him to identify the direction of each movement. Before you do this, ensure that the patient does not have any pain in the fingers, for example, from osteoarthritis.

▶ **Vibration.** Apply a vibrating 128 Hz tuning fork first over the sternum and then over the bony prominences of the upper arm. Compare both sides.

After the examination

Thank the patient.

Ask to carry out a full neurological examination.

Summarise your findings and offer a differential diagnosis.

Most common conditions likely to come up in an *Examine the sensory system of the upper limbs* OSCE:

- Mononeuropathy.
- Radiculopathy.
- Cortical lesion.

28. Examine the motor system of the upper limbs

Before starting

Introduce yourself to the patient.

Explain the examination and ask for his permission to carry it out.

Position him and ask him to expose his upper limbs.

The examination

Inspection

○ Look for any abnormal posturing.

○ Look for any abnormal movements such as fasciculation, tremor, dystonia or athetosis.

○ Assess the muscles of the hands, arms and shoulder girdle for size, shape and symmetry. You can also measure the circumference of the arms.

Tone

○ Ensure that the patient is not in any pain.

○ Test the tone in the upper limbs by holding the patient's hand and simultaneously pronating and supinating and flexing and extending the forearm. If you suspect increased tone, ask the patient to clench his teeth and re-test. Is the increased tone best described as spasticity (clasp-knife) or as rigidity (lead pipe)? Spasticity suggests a pyramidal lesion, rigidity suggests an extra-pyramidal lesion.

Power

○ Test muscle strength for shoulder abduction, elbow flexion and extension, wrist flexion and extension, finger flexion, extension, and abduction, and thumb abduction. Compare muscle strength on both sides, and grade it on the MRC muscle strength scale:

- 0 No movement.
- 1 Feeble contractions.
- 2 Movement.
- 3 Movement against gravity.
- 4 Movement against resistance.
- 5 Full strength.

Important root values in the upper limb	
Shoulder abduction (deltoid)	C5
Elbow flexion	C6
Elbow extension	C7
Finger flexion	C8
Finger abduction	T1

Reflexes

▷ Test the biceps, supinator and triceps reflexes with a tendon hammer. Compare both sides. If a reflex cannot be elicited, ask the patient to clench his teeth and re-test.

Spinal roots tested by reflexes	
Reflex	**Spinal root(s)**
Biceps	C5, C6
Supinator	C6
Triceps	C7

Cerebellar signs

▷ Test for intention tremor, dysynergia, and dysmetria by asking the patient to alternately touch his nose and then your finger (the finger-to-nose test). Ask him to do it as fast as possible.

▷ Then test for dysdiadochokinesis by asking him to clap one hand against the other, simultaneously pronating and supinating it. Ask him to do this as fast as possible.

After the examination

Thank the patient.

Ask to carry out a full neurological examination.

Summarise your findings and offer a differential diagnosis.

Most common conditions likely to come up in an *Examine the motor system of the upper limbs* OSCE:

▷ Parkinson's disease.

▷ Cerebellar syndrome.

▷ Ulnar, median or radial nerve lesion.

▷ Radiculopathy.

▷ Myopathy.

▷ Hemiplegia.

29. Examine the sensory system of the lower limbs

Before starting

Introduce yourself to the patient.

Explain the examination and ask for his permission to carry it out.

Position him and ask him to expose his legs.

The examination

To examine the sensory system, test light touch, pain, proprioception and vibration sense. Don't forget to inspect the legs before you start.

▶ **Light touch.** Ask the patient to close his eyes and apply a wisp of cotton or tissue to the sternum and then to each of the dermatomes of the leg. Compare both sides.

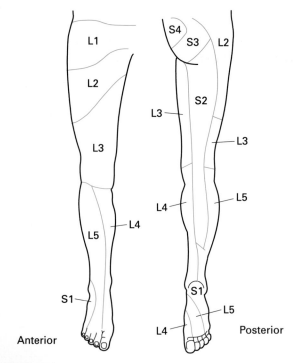

Figure 5. Dermatomes of the leg

▶ **Pain.** Ask the patient to close his eyes and apply a sharp object – ideally a neurological pin – to the sternum and then to each of the dermatomes of the leg. Compare both sides.

○ Proprioception. Ask the patient to close his eyes. Hold one of the toes by its sides and move it at the interphalangeal joint, asking him to identify the direction of each movement. Before you do this, ensure that the patient does not have any pain in the toes, from osteoarthritis, for example. If the patient can stand, you can also perform Romberg's test (see Chapter 26, *Examine gait and co-ordination*).

○ Vibration. Apply a vibrating 128 Hz tuning fork first over the sternum and then over the bony prominences of the legs. Compare both sides.

After the examination

Thank the patient.

Ask to carry out a full neurological examination.

Summarise your findings and offer a differential diagnosis.

Most common conditions likely to come up in an *Examine the sensory system of the lower limbs* OSCE:

○ Peripheral neuropathy.

○ Mononeuropathy.

○ Cortical lesion.

○ Cauda equina lesion.

○ Radiculopathy.

30. Examine the motor system of the lower limbs

Before starting

Introduce yourself to the patient.

Explain the examination and ask for his consent to carry it out.

Position him and ask him to expose his legs.

The examination

Inspection

▶ Look for deformities of the foot.

▶ Look for abnormal posturing.

▶ Look for fasciculation.

▶ Assess the muscles of the legs for size, shape and symmetry. You can also measure the circumference of the quadriceps or calves.

Tone

▶ Ensure that the patient is not in any pain.

▶ Test the tone in the legs by rolling the leg on the bed, by flexing and extending the knee or by abruptly lifting the leg at the knee.

Power

▶ Test muscle strength for hip flexion, extension, abduction and adduction, knee flexion and extension, and plantar flexion and dorsiflexion of the foot and big toe. Compare muscle strength on both sides, and grade it on the MRC muscle strength scale:

0   No movement.
1   Feeble contractions.
2   Movement.
3   Movement against gravity.
4   Movement against resistance.
5   Full strength.

Important root values in the lower limb	
Hip flexion	L1
Hip adduction	L2
Knee extension	L3
Foot dorsiflexion	L4
Big toe dorsiflexion	L5
Foot plantar flexion	S1

Reflexes

▶ Test the knee jerk and ankle jerk using a tendon hammer. Compare both sides. If a reflex cannot be elicited, ask the patient to clench his teeth and re-test.

Spinal roots tested by reflexes	
Reflex	Spinal root(s)
Knee jerk	L3, L4
Ankle jerk	L5, S1

▶ Test for clonus by dorsiflexing the foot.

▶ Test for the Babinsky sign (extensor plantar reflex) using the sharp end of the tendon hammer.

Cerebellar signs

▶ Heel-knee-shin test: Ask the patient to bring his ankle onto his knee and to slide it down his shin. Test both legs.

Gait

▶ If he can, ask the patient to walk five or so paces and then to turn around and walk back. (See Chapter 26, *Examine gait and co-ordination*).

After the examination

Thank the patient.

Ask to carry out a full neurological examination.

Summarise your findings and offer a differential diagnosis.

Most common conditions likely to come up in an *Examine the motor system of the lower limbs* OSCE:

▶ Radiculopathy.

▶ Peripheral neuropathy.

▶ Hemiplegia.

▶ Cauda equina lesion.

▶ Myopathy.

31. Take a general psychiatric history

Specifications: This is usually a double station, so as to give you more time.

! For this station, it is especially important to put the patient at ease, and to be seen to be sensitive, tactful and empathic.

Before starting

Introduce yourself to the patient.

Ensure that he is comfortable. Before starting, it is a good idea to make some general comments to put him at ease.

The history

○ Name, age and occupation.

Presenting complaint

○ Ask mainly open questions and listen carefully to the patient.

○ Determine the mode of referral.

History of presenting complaint

Ask about:

○ The onset and duration of the symptoms.

○ The effect the symptoms are having on the patient's everyday life.

○ Any treatment so far.

○ Previous episodes of the illness.

○ Previous treatments and their outcome.

Ask screening questions about mood, phobias and obsessions, abnormal experiences, and abnormal beliefs. (See Chapter 32, *Assess mental state*).

Informant history

If the patient is accompanied by a relative, friend or carer, an informant history should be taken at this stage.

Past psychiatric history

○ Previous admissions, formal or informal.

○ History of violence.

○ Past suicide attempts.

Past medical history

- Current illness:
    - Acute illness.
    - Chronic illness.
    - Vascular risk factors.
- Past and childhood illnesses.
- Surgery.
- Recent visits to the doctor.

Drug history

- Prescribed medication.
- Recent changes in prescribed medication.
- Over-the-counter drugs.
- Allergies.

Family history

- Determine if anyone in the family has suffered from similar problems.
- Has anyone in the family ever tried to kill themselves?

Personal history

Aim to cover:

- Birth.
- Developmental milestones.
- Educational achievement.
- Occupational history.
- Drugs and alcohol: pattern of misuse, symptoms of dependence, social ramifications.
- Forensic history.
- Psychosexual history: partners, quality of relationship, children, homosexuality.
- Religious orientation.

Social history

- Housing.
- Family and social support.
- Self-care.
- Typical day.
- Interests and hobbies.
- Finances.

After taking the history

Ask the patient if there is anything he might add that you have forgotten to ask about.

Summarise your findings and offer a differential diagnosis.

Thank the patient.

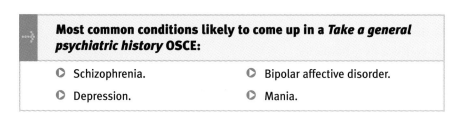

Most common conditions likely to come up in a *Take a general psychiatric history* OSCE:

- Schizophrenia.
- Bipolar affective disorder.
- Depression.
- Mania.

32. Assess mental state

Specifications: This is usually a double station, so as to give you more time. You are usually not required to include a cognitive assessment.

Before starting

Introduce yourself to the patient.

Explain that you would like to explore his thoughts, and ask him if this is OK.

Take out a pen and pad!

Assessing the mental state

The mental state can be assessed under eight main headings:

- Appearance and behaviour
- Speech
- Mood
- Phobias and obsessions
- Abnormal experiences
- Abnormal beliefs
- Insight
- Cognition

Begin by asking the patient some open questions, focusing your attention on the patient's *appearance and behaviour*.

- Appearance: dress, posture, facial expression, mannerisms.
- Activity.
- Social and emotional behaviour: apathy, irritability, lability, general co-operativity.
- Presence of catatonic features.

Also focus on his *speech*.

- Rate.
- Tone.
- Quality.
- Form: thought block, loosening of associations, flight of ideas, perseverations/echolalia, neologisms, clang associations.
- Content, e.g., depressive ideas, ruminations, delusions.

Then ask specifically about:

Mood

- Anxiety symptoms: subjective feeling of anxiety, sweating, palpitations, breathlessness, paraesthesia.
- Current mood state and severity.

! **Determine both the subjective and the objective state of mood. Depression should trigger a range of questions (see *Interview a patient with depression*, Chapter 33).**

- ▷ Biological symptoms: sleep, appetite, libido, lack of energy.
- ▷ Suicidal ideas: *Have you ever thought of killing yourself?*

Phobias and obsessions

- ▷ Phobias: for a phobia, determine the stimulus, its psychological and physiological effect, and the nature of any avoidance behaviour; does the patient suffer from the General Anxiety Syndrome (GAS)?
- ▷ Obsessions: for an obsession, determine the underlying fear, the nature of any resistance and the effect of the obsession on daily life. Is the obsession perceived as being senseless?

Abnormal experiences

- ▷ Depersonalisation.
- ▷ Derealisation.
- ▷ Illusions/misperceptions.
- ▷ Hallucinations (modality, content, mood congruency). For auditory hallucinations, is there more than one voice, and do the voices talk *to* the patient (second person) or *about* the patient (third person)?

Abnormal beliefs

- ▷ Overvalued ideas.
- ▷ Delusions.

Insight

To determine the level of insight, ask the patient:

- ▷ *What do you think is wrong with you?*
- ▷ *Do you think you need treatment?*
- ▷ *What are you hoping the treatment will do for you?*

Cognition

To assess cognition, perform the Mini Mental State Examination.

After assessing the mental state

Thank the patient.

Summarise your findings.

Offer a differential diagnosis.

> **Most common conditions likely to come up in an *Assess mental state* OSCE:**
>
> - Depression.
> - Schizophrenia.
> - Mania.
> - Bipolar affective disorder.
> - Obsessive compulsive disorder.

33. Interview a patient with depression

! **For this station, it is especially important to put the patient at ease, and to be sensitive, tactful, and empathic.**

Before starting

Introduce yourself to the patient.

Explain that you are going to ask him some questions to uncover exactly how he is feeling, and ask for his consent to do this.

Ensure that he is comfortable.

Ask for his name, age and occupation.

The interview

○ First ask an open question or open questions about the patient's current mood and feelings, listening attentively and gently encouraging the patient to open up.

○ Ask about the onset of illness, and about its triggers or causes.

Ensure that you ask about:

○ The *core features* of depression:
  ○ Depressed mood.
  ○ Loss of interest.
  ○ Fatiguability.

○ Other *common features* of depression:
  ○ Reduced concentration.
  ○ Poor self-esteem.
  ○ Guilt.
  ○ Pessimism.
  ○ Sleep disturbance.
  ○ Loss of appetite.
  ○ Loss of libido.

○ The *somatic features* of depression:
  ○ Anhedonia.
  ○ Early morning waking.
  ○ Morning depression.
  ○ Agitation and retardation.

▶ Ask about hallucinations, delusions and mania, to exclude other possible psychiatric diagnoses.

▶ Take brief past medical, drug and family histories.

▶ Assess the severity of the illness and the effect on the patient's life.

▶ Ask about suicidal intent. If the patient is suicidal, assess suicidal intent. (See Chapter 34, *Assess suicidal intent*).

Before finishing

Ask the patient if there is anything he might add that you have forgotten to ask about.

Thank the patient and offer a further course of action (e.g., refer to the GP).

34. Assess suicidal intent

Introduce yourself to the patient.

Establish rapport.

Ask about:

- The history of the current episode of self-harm (if any):
  - What was the precipitant for the attempt?
  - Was it planned?
  - What was the method of self-harm?
  - Did the patient leave a suicide note?
  - Was he alone?
  - Was he intoxicated?
  - Did he take any precautions against discovery?
  - Did he seek help after the attempt?
- Assess risk factors for suicide:
  - Male sex.
  - Age > 45.
  - Unemployed.
  - Isolated.
  - Divorced, widowed or single.
  - Physical illness.
  - Psychiatric illness.
  - Substance misuse.
  - Previous suicide attempts.
  - Family history of depression, substance misuse and suicide.
- Assess current mood. In particular, ask about depression and anger.
- Will the patient be returning to the same situation?
- What is the patient's outlook on the future?
- Ask about current suicidal ideation. Has the patient made any plans?

Thank the patient.

Summarise your findings, state the patient's suicide risk and suggest a plan of action (e.g., psychiatric evaluation, hospitalisation...).

35. Interview a patient with anorexia

Introduce yourself to the patient.

Explain that you are going to ask her some questions about her eating habits, and ask for her consent to do this.

Ensure that she is comfortable.

Ask for her name, age, and occupation.

The interview

Weight

Determine:

- Her current weight.
- The amount of weight that she has lost, and over how long.
- Whether the weight loss has been intentional.
- Whether she still considers herself to be overweight.

Diet

Ask about:

- Amount and type of food eaten in an average day.
- Binge eating.
- Vomiting.
- The use of laxatives, purgatives or diuretics.

Other

Ask about:

- Menstruation.
- Depression.
- Previous treatment for anorexia.
- Investigations for medical causes of weight loss such as thyroid disease or Crohn's disease.
- Past medical, drug and family history (briefly).
- Social history.

Before finishing

Ask the patient if there is anything she might add that you have forgotten to ask about.

Determine the patient's level of insight into her problem.

Thank the patient, offer feedback and suggest a further course of action, e.g. investigations, psychotherapy, hospitalisation.

Ask to take a collateral history from the patient's mother.

36. Take an alcohol history

Before starting

Introduce yourself to the patient.

Establish rapport.

Explain to the patient that you would like to ask him some questions to evaluate his drinking habits, and ask for his consent to do this.

The alcohol history

Ask about

- Alcohol intake:
  - Amount.
  - Type.
  - Place.
  - Time.
- Features of alcohol dependence:
  - Compulsion to drink.
  - Increased tolerance to alcohol.
  - Narrowing of drinking repertoire.
- Withdrawal symptoms:
  - Anxiety.
  - Tremor.
  - Sweating.
  - Nausea.
  - Fits.
  - Hallucinations.

Symptoms typically occur after a period of abstinence, for example, first thing in the morning, and are relieved by alcohol.

Medical history

- Focus on the medical complications of alcohol abuse, e.g., peptic ulceration, pancreatitis, ischaemic heart disease, liver disease, peripheral neuropathy.

Drug history

- Alcohol potentiates the effects of certain drugs such as phenytoin.

Social history

- Employment.
- Marital problems.
- Financial problems.
- Legal problems.

Family history

- Alcohol abuse.

After taking the alcohol history

Give the patient feedback on his drinking habits.

Suggest ways for him to reduce his alcohol consumption, if appropriate.

Ask him if he has any questions or concerns.

Thank him for his co-operation.

37. Examine hearing and the ear

Before starting

Introduce yourself to the patient.

Explain the examination and ask for his consent to carry it out.

Sit him so that he is facing you and ensure that he is comfortable.

The history

▷ Name and age.

Ask the patient if there has been any loss of hearing.

If there has been loss of hearing, assess its:

▷ Characteristics (bilaterality, onset, duration, severity, impact on patient's life).

▷ Associated features.

▷ Possible causes.

The examination

Hearing

Test hearing by whispering into an ear at various distances, whilst distracting or occluding the other ear.

Tuning fork tests

! Use a 512 Hz tuning fork, and not the 256 Hz fork that is used for neurological examinations.

▷ The Rinne test: Place the base of the vibrating tuning fork on the mastoid process of each ear. Once the patient can no longer "hear" the vibration, move the tuning fork in front of the ear. If the tuning fork can be heard, air conduction is better than bone conduction, and there is therefore no conductive hearing loss. The test is said to be *positive*. If the tuning fork cannot be heard, there is a conductive hearing loss, and the test is said to be *negative*.

! The false negative Rinne test: If the Rinne test is performed on a deaf ear, it may appear negative because the vibration is transmitted to the opposite ear.

▷ The Weber test: Place the vibrating tuning fork in the midline of the skull. If hearing is normal, or if hearing loss is symmetrical, the vibration should be heard equally in both ears.

Note:

- ▷ If there is conductive deafness in one ear, the vibration is best heard *in that same ear.*
- ▷ If there is sensorineural deafness in one ear, the vibration is best heard in the other ear.

Auroscopy

- ▷ Examine the pinnae for size, shape, deformities, pre-auricular sinuses.
- ▷ Look behind the ears for any scars.
- ▷ Palpate the pre-auricular, post-auricular and infra-auricular lymph nodes.
- ▷ Affix a speculum of appropriate size onto the auroscope.
- ▷ Gently pull the ear so as to straighten the ear canal and, holding the auroscope like a pen, introduce it into the external auditory meatus.

If examining the right ear, use your right hand to hold the auroscope. If examining the left ear, use your left hand.

- ▷ Inspect the ear canal (otitis externa, exotoses, wax) and the tympanic membrane (normal anatomy, effusions, cholesteatomata, perforations, grommets).

After examining the ear

Thank the patient.

Summarise your findings and offer a differential diagnosis.

38. Examine vision and the eye

Before starting

Introduce yourself to the patient.

Explain the examination and ask for his consent to carry it out.

Ensure that he is comfortable.

The examination

Visual acuity

○ *Snellen chart*. Assess each eye individually, correcting for any refractive errors (glasses, pinhole). If the patient cannot read the Snellen chart, either move him closer or ask him to count fingers. If he fails to count fingers, test whether he can see hand movements and, if he cannot, test whether he can see light.

○ *Test types* (or fine print). Again, assess each eye individually, correcting for any refractive errors.

○ *Ishihara plates*. Indicate that you could use Ishihara plates to test colour vision specifically.

Visual fields

○ *Confrontation test*. Sit at 1 m from the patient. Cover your right eye and ask the patient to cover his left eye and to fix his right eye on your left eye. Starting at a distance, bring a moving finger into each of the four quadrants of the visual field, comparing the patient's visual field to your own. Test the other eye.

○ *Visual inattention test*. Simultaneously bring a moving finger into each of the patient's right and left visual fields. In some parietal lobe lesions, only the ipsilateral finger is perceived by the patient.

○ *Mapping of central visual field defects*. Indicate that you could use a red pin to delineate the patient's blind spot and any central visual field defects.

Pupillary reflexes

○ *Inspection*. Inspect the pupils for size and shape.

○ *Pupillary reflexes*. Ask the patient to fixate on a distant object and, using a pen torch, test the direct and consensual pupillary reflexes. If the consensual pupillary reflex is absent, there is a relative afferent pupillary defect, or Marcus Gunn pupil.

○ *Accommodation reflex*. Test the accommodation reflex by asking the patient to focus on a distant object and then on a finger held at 30 cm from his face.

Eye movements

○ *Inspection*. Look for a squint.

○ *Cover test*. Indicate that you could perform a cover test to look for a concomitant squint.

○ *Eye movements*. Fix the patient's head and ask him to track your finger through an "H" pattern. Ask him to report any diplopia.

○ *Nystagmus*.

Fundoscopy

Darken the room and ask the patient to fixate on a distant object (or to "look over my shoulder").

○ *Red reflex*. Test from a distance of 1m. An absent red reflex is usually caused by a cataract.

○ *Fundoscopy*. Use your right eye to examine the patient's right eye, and your left eye to examine the patient's left eye. If you use your left eye to examine the patient's right eye, you will appear more caring than the examiner might like to see. Look at the optic nerve, the vessels and the macula.

After the examination

Thank the patient.

Summarise your findings and offer a differential diagnosis.

39. Examine the neck

Before starting

Introduce yourself to the patient.

Explain the examination and ask for his consent to carry it out.

Ask him to expose the neck and upper body.

Sit him in a chair.

The examination

Inspection

- Inspect the patient generally, in particular looking for any signs of thyroid disease. The age and sex of the patient can influence the differential diagnosis of a goitre.

- Inspect the neck, looking for asymmetry, scars or other lesions.

! **A goitre, or enlarged thyroid gland, is seen as a swelling below the cricoid cartilage, on either side of the trachea.**

- Ask the patient to take a sip of water. Only a goitre, a thyroglossal cyst and lymph nodes move on swallowing.

- Ask the patient to stick his tongue out. A midline swelling which moves upwards when the tongue is protruded is a thyroglossal cyst.

Palpation

- Position yourself behind the patient.

- Ask the patient if he has any tenderness in the neck.

- Putting one hand on either side of the patient's neck, examine the anterior and posterior triangles of the neck. For any mass, try to determine its size, consistency and fixity.

- Palpate the thyroid gland. Try to determine its size, symmetry and consistency, and if it is tender to touch. Note that the normal thyroid gland is often not palpable.

- Palpate the cervical lymph nodes.

- Palpate for tracheal deviation in the suprasternal notch (see Chapter 15, *Examine the respiratory system*).

Percussion

- Percuss for the dullness of a retrosternal goitre over the sternum and upper chest.

Auscultation

- Auscultate over the thyroid for bruits. Ask the patient to hold his breath as you listen: a soft bruit is sometimes heard in thyrotoxicosis.

After the examination

Help the patient to put his clothes back on.

Ask the patient is he has any questions or concerns.

Thank the patient.

Offer a diagnosis or differential diagnosis.

Give suggestions for further management, e.g., thyroid function tests, thyroid antibodies, ultrasound examination of the thyroid, iodine thyroid scan, fine-needle aspiration cytology.

Key signs of thyroid disease

- Thyrotoxicosis: enlarged thyroid gland or thyroid nodules, thyroid bruit, sympathetic signs such as tremor and tachycardia, onycholysis.

    - Graves disease: uniformly enlarged smooth thyroid gland usually in a younger patient; exophthalmos, pre-tibial myxoedema, thyroid acropachy.

    - Toxic multinodular goitre: enlarged multinodular goitre in a middle-aged patient.

- Hashimoto's thyroiditis: moderately enlarged rubbery thyroid gland, usually in a female patient of age 30–50; initial hyperthryroidism that progresses to hypothyroidism and, if untreated, to myxoedema.

Most common conditions likely to come up in an *Examine the neck* OSCE:

- Thyroglossal cyst.

- Toxic goitre: diffuse (Grave's disease), multinodular, toxic nodule (Plummer's disease).

- Hashimoto's thyroiditis.

- Thyroid neoplasm.

- Enlarged lymph node(s).

- Physiological goitre of puberty or of pregnancy (or of both, these days).

40. Take a history from a parent and child

Taking a history from a parent and child is a fine art and one that requires practice. Do not forget that you are interviewing two people and that both their concerns must be met. As a rule of thumb, the older the child, the more he should be involved.

Although the structure of the paediatric history is the same as that of any other history, there are some important extra questions that should be asked.

Finally don't forget to observe the child, as important clues can be gained from doing this.

Before starting

Introduce yourself to the parent and to the child.

Explain that you are going to ask some questions and obtain consent to do this.

Ensure that the patient is comfortable; younger children may need toys to keep them distracted.

The history

- Ask the age, sex and preferred name of the child.
- Confirm the relationship of the accompanying adult.

Presenting complaint and history of presenting complaint

- Ask about the nature of the presenting complaint and how it has affected the child's daily routine. Start by using open questions and then explore the symptoms as you might in any other history.

! **Do not, under any circumstances, omit to address, or denigrate, the parent's concerns.**

Systems review

- The major systems should be covered briefly, putting the emphasis on areas of particular relevance:
  - *General Health*: Liveliness, change in behaviour.
  - *CVS and RS*: Breathing problems (feeding in young infants), cyanosis, cough, tiredness.
  - *GIS*: Feeding, nutrition, vomiting, diarrhoea/constipation, abdominal pain.
  - *GUS*: Frequency, discharge, enuresis.
  - *NS*: Headaches, visual disturbances, fits.
  - *MSS*: Limps.

Past medical history

Ask about these topics if you think that they might be relevant to the child's presenting complaint.

- Birth history
  - Maternal obstetric history.
  - Mode of delivery.
  - Gestation.
  - Birth weight.
  - Admission to Special Care Baby Unit.
- Developmental milestones. (See Chapter 41, *Perform a developmental assessment*).
- Immunisations.
- Childhood illnesses/visits to the doctor.
- Education.
- Nutrition.

Drug history

- Prescribed and over-the-counter drugs.
- Allergies.

Family history

- Congenital/genetic abnormalities ("Are there any illnesses that run in the family?").
- Cosanguinity.
- Health of parents and siblings.

Social history

- Parental occupation.
- Details of home life, siblings.
- Behaviour at home and at school.

After taking the history

Ask the parent if there is anything that he might add that you have forgotten to ask.

Ask the parent and child if they have any specific questions or concerns.

Thank the parent and child.

Summarise your findings and offer a differential diagnosis.

Most common conditions likely to come up in a *Take a history from a parent and child* OSCE:

- Respiratory conditions, e.g., asthma, upper respiratory tract infections.

- Headaches.

- Behavioural problems: Autism, nocturnal enuresis.

- Fits, e.g., febrile convulsions, epilepsy.

- Childhood infections/rashes and immunisation compliance (see Chapter 49, *Child immunisation programme*).

41. Perform a developmental assessment

Development in the early years of life is fairly consistent from child to child and any significant deviation from this pattern is thus a reliable marker of pathology.

The four parameters used in assessing development:

1. Motor skills
2. Vision and fine movement
3. Hearing and language
4. Social behaviour

Key ages for developmental assessment:

1. Newborn
2. Supine infant (1.5–2 months)
3. Sitting infant (6–9 months)
4. Toddler (18–24 months)
5. Communicating child (3–4 years)

Average ages for the acquisition of key milestones				
	Motor skills	**Vision and fine movement**	**Hearing and language**	**Social behaviour**
Newborn	Symmetrical movements, limbs flexed	Looks at light/ faces	Responds to noises/voices	Responds to parents
Supine infant	Raises head when prone	Follows objects	Normal cry	Smiles
Sitting infant	6 months: Sits 9 months: Stands with support	6 months: Palmar grasp 7 months: Transfers	Babbles	Finger feeds
Toddler	12 months: Walks 24 months: Climbs stairs	12 months: Pincer grip	12 months: 1–3 words 24 months: Phrases	12 months: Drinks from cup 24 months: Undresses
Communicating child	Pedals tricycle	Mature pencil grip	Uses complete sentences	Plays with other children

The developmental assessment

The developmental assessment is usually performed alongside a general history, so many of the subject headings are the same as in Chapter 40, *Take a history from a parent and child*. Remember to tailor the assessment to the age of the child and to observe the child's behaviour at all times.

Before starting

Introduce yourself to the parent and child.

Explain that you are going to ask some questions and obtain consent to do this.

Ensure that the patient is comfortable; younger children may need toys to keep them distracted.

The assessment

○ Ask the age, sex and preferred name of the child.

Presenting complaint and history of presenting complaint

Ask about the nature of the presenting complaint and its effect on the child's daily routine. Use open questions.

Developmental/Past medical history

○ Birth history:

   ○ Maternal obstetric history.

   ○ Delivery.

   ○ Gestation.

   ○ Birth weight.

   ○ Admission to Special Care Baby Unit.

   ○ Initial feeding.

○ Milestones:

   ○ Smiling.

   ○ Sitting.

   ○ Walking.

   ○ Talking.

○ Current abilities:

Cover:

   ○ Motor skills.

   ○ Vision and fine movement.

   ○ Language and hearing.

   ○ Social behaviour.

- Childhood illnesses/visits to the doctor.
- Immunisation history.
- Education.
- Nutrition.

Systems review

Drug history

Family history

Social history

After the assessment

Ask the parent if there is anything they might add that you have forgotten to ask.

Ask the parent/child if they have any specific questions or concerns.

Thank the patient.

Summarise your findings and offer a differential diagnosis.

Most common conditions likely to come up in a *Perform a developmental assessment* OSCE:

- Late walker.
- Cerebral palsy.
- Mental handicap (chromosomal abnormalities).
- Autism.

42. Perform a neonatal examination

Specifications: A mannequin in lieu of a baby. The baby's "mother" is also in the room.

Before starting

Wash your hands.

Ask the mother about:

- Any complications of the pregnancy.
- Type of delivery.
- The baby's gestational age at the time of birth.
- The baby's birth weight.
- The baby's feeding, urination and defecation.
- Any concerns that she might have.

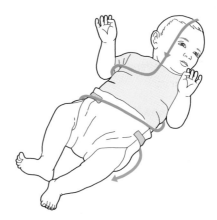

Figure 6. General order of examination

The examination

General inspection

Note colour, position, tone and any obvious abnormalities.

Head

- Palpate the fontanelles.
- Measure the head circumference.

Face

Check for:

- The patency of the ears.
- The patency of the nostrils.
- The red reflex, pupillary reflexes and eye movements (squints).
- Introduce a finger into the baby's mouth and feel the palate (cleft palate).
- Examine the palate using a torch and spatula.

Chest

- Take the radial and femoral pulses, one after another and then both at the same time (radiofemoral delay).
- Listen to the heart using the bell of your stethoscope.
- Listen to the lungs using the diaphragm of your stethoscope. Turn the infant over to listen on the back.

Back

- Examine the spine, focusing on the sacral pit.
- Check the patency of the anus.

Abdomen

- Inspect the abdomen and the umbilical cord.
- Palpate the abdomen generally.
- Palpate specifically for the spleen, liver, and kidneys (thumb in front, finger in loin).
- Examine the genitalia. In male infants note the position of the urethra, ask about the urine stream and feel for the testicles.

Hips

- Abduct the hips (Ortolani test).
- Next, adduct them applying pressure on your thumbs (Barlow's test).

Arms and hands

- Inspect the arms and hands, paying particular attention to the palmar creases.

Feet

- Inspect the feet and test their range of movement.

Posture and reflexes

▷ Pick up the baby by the arms to test head lag.

▷ Hold the baby prone – his head should lie above the midline.

▷ Test the Moro reflex by lifting the head and shoulders and then suddenly dropping them back – the arms should abduct and extend in a symmetrical fashion.

▷ Test the grasp reflex by placing your finger in the baby's hand.

▷ Test the knee jerk and the Babinski (extensor plantar) reflex.

After the neonatal examination

Summarise your findings.

Reassure the mother, or tell her that you are going to have the baby examined by a senior colleague.

43. Perform a six-week check

Specifications: A mannequin in lieu of a baby.

Before starting

Introduce yourself to the parent.

Explain the nature of the examination and ensure consent.

Ask for the parent-held record.

The history

▷ Ask the exact age, sex and preferred name of the child.

Main concerns

▷ Ask if the parent has any specific concerns, as these need to be addressed.

Past medical history

▷ Birth history:

- ▷ Pregnancy.
- ▷ Gestation.
- ▷ Delivery.
- ▷ Birth weight.
- ▷ Neonatal history.

Present health

▷ Current health status.

▷ Medication.

▷ Social history.

The examination

PART 1 – DEVELOPMENTAL ASSESSMENT

Motor skills

▷ Symmetrical limb movements.

▷ Head lag.

Vision and fine movement

▷ Looks at light/faces.

▷ Follows an object.

Hearing and language

- Responds to noises/voices.
- Normal cry.
- Ask parent if he/she is concerned about the baby's hearing.

Social behaviour

- Smiles responsively.

PART 2 – PHYSICAL EXAMINATION

Growth

- Weight.
- Length.
- Head circumference.
- Plot findings on a centile chart.

Head

- Palpate the fontanelles.

Face

- Eyes: red reflex, pupillary reflexes and eye movements (squints).
- Ears.
- Mouth. Use a pen torch.

Chest

- Feel for the radial and femoral pulses.
- Auscultate over the heart.
- Auscultate over the lungs.

Back

- Examine the spine, particularly the sacral pit.

Abdomen

- Inspect and palpate the abdomen.
- Examine the external genitalia.

Hips

▶ Abduct the hips (Ortolani test).

▶ Next, adduct them applying pressure on your thumbs (Barlow's test).

After the surveillance review

Discuss your findings with the parent.

Use this opportunity for health promotion, e.g., immunisations, accident prevention, detecting hearing problems, services available for the parents of young children.

Elicit any remaining concerns that the parent might have.

Thank the parent.

44. Paediatric examination: cardiovascular system

It is unlikely that you should be asked to examine the cardiovascular system of a younger child. If this should happen, be prepared to change the order of the examination and modify your technique as appropriate. For example, you may have to examine the child on the parent's knee or listen to the chest before the child starts crying.

Before starting

Introduce yourself to the child and the parent.

Tell the child that you are going to examine his chest.

Position him at 45 degrees, and ask him to remove his top(s).

Ensure that he is comfortable.

The examination

General inspection

○ Observe the child carefully, looking for any obvious abnormalities in his general appearance.

! Don't be afraid to state the obvious.

○ Does the child look his age? (Mention the growth chart).

○ Is he breathless or cyanosed?

○ Inspect the precordium and the chest for any scars and pulsations. A median sternotomy or thoracotomy scar might indicate the repair of a congenital heart defect such as a patent ductus arteriosus or a ventricular septal defect.

Inspection and examination of the hands

○ Take both hands and assess them for:

  ○ Colour and temperature.

  ○ Clubbing.

  ○ Splinter haemorrhages.

  ○ Nail signs.

○ Determine the rate, rhythm and character of the radial pulse (brachial pulse in younger infants). Take the femoral pulse at the same time to exclude a coarctation of the aorta.

Normal pulse rates in children	
Age in years	Pulse (beats/min)
< 1	100–160
2–4	90–140
4–10	80–140
> 10	65–100

▷ Indicate that you would like to record the blood pressure. Remember to use a cuff of an appropriate size.

Inspection and examination of the head and neck

▷ Inspect the sclera for signs of anaemia.

▷ Inspect the mouth and tongue for signs of central cyanosis.

▷ Assess the jugular venous pressure (difficult in very young infants).

▷ Locate the carotid pulse and assess its character.

Palpation of the heart

! Ask the child if he has any chest pain.

▷ Determine the location and character of the apex beat. In children (up to 8 years), this is found at the fourth intercostal space in the mid-clavicular line.

▷ Palpate the precordium. Remember that a thrill is simply a palpable murmur.

Auscultation of the heart

! Warm the diaphragm of your stethoscope.

▷ Listen for heart sounds, additional sounds and murmurs. Using the stethoscope's diaphragm, listen in:

  ▷ The *aortic* area.
  ▷ The *pulmonary* area.
  ▷ The *tricuspid* area.
  ▷ The *mitral* area.

▷ Any murmur must be classified according to:

  ▷ Timing.
  ▷ Grade.
  ▷ Site.
  ▷ Radiation.

> ### Innocent murmurs are common in childhood
>
> An innocent murmur is:
>
> - Systolic.
> - Low grade.
> - Heard over a small area.
> - Asymptomatic.

Chest examination

Auscultate the chest, especially at the bases of the lungs.

Abdominal examination

Palpate the abdomen to exclude ascites and/or an enlarged liver. The liver edge can usually be palpated in younger infants.

Peripheral pulses

Feel the temperature of the feet and palpate the femoral pulses.

After the examination

Cover the child.

Thank the child and parent.

Summarise your findings and offer a differential diagnosis.

> ### Most common conditions likely to come up in a *Paediatric examination: cardiovascular system* OSCE:
>
> - Ventricular septal defect: loud pan-systolic murmur (=small VSD).
> - Patent ductus arteriosus: continuous, loud, machine-like murmur that radiates to the back.
> - Atrial septal defect: ejection systolic murmur.
> - Pulmonary stenosis: ejection systolic murmur.
> - Aortic stenosis/Hypertrophic obstructive cardiomyopathy: ejection systolic murmur.
> - Coarctation of the aorta.

45. Paediatric examination: respiratory system

It is unlikely that you should be asked to examine the respiratory system of a younger child. If this should happen, be prepared to change the order of the examination and modify your technique as appropriate.

Before starting

Introduce yourself to the child and the parent.

Tell the child that you are going to examine his chest.

Position him at 45 degrees, and ask him to remove his top(s).

Ensure that he is comfortable.

The examination

General inspection

Observe the child carefully, looking for any obvious abnormalities in his general appearance.

! **Don't be afraid to state the obvious.**

- Does the child look his age? (Mention the growth chart).
- Is he breathless or cyanosed?
- Is his breathing audible?
- Note the rate, depth and regularity of his breathing.
- Look around the child for other clues such as a PEFR meter, inhalers, etc.

Normal respiratory rates in children	
Age	**Respiratory rate (breaths/min)**
Premature infant	40–60
Term infant	30–50
6 years	19–24
12 years	16–21

Look for:

- Deformities of the chest (barrel chest, pectus excavatum, pectus carinatum) and spine.
- Asymmetry of chest expansion.
- The use of accessory muscles of respiration.
- Harrison's sulci.
- Operative scars.

Inspection and examination of the hands

○ Take both hands and assess them for colour and temperature.

○ Look for clubbing.

○ Determine the rate, rhythm, and character of the radial pulse (brachial pulse in younger infants).

Inspection and examination of head and neck

○ Inspect the sclera for signs of anaemia.

○ Inspect the mouth for signs of central cyanosis.

○ Assess the jugular venous pressure and the jugular venous pulse form.

○ Palpate the cervical, supraclavicular, infraclavicular and axillary lymph nodes.

Palpation of the chest

! Ask the child if he has any chest pain.

○ Palpate for tracheal deviation by placing the index and middle fingers of one hand on either side of the trachea in the suprasternal notch. (This can be omitted in younger children as it may cause discomfort).

○ Palpate for the position of the cardiac apex.

Note: Carry out all subsequent steps on the front of the chest and, once this is done, repeat them on the back of the chest.

○ Palpate for equal chest expansion, comparing one side to the other.

○ Palpate for tactile fremitus.

Percussion of the chest

○ Percuss the chest. (Not useful in young infants). Start at the apex of one lung, and compare one side to the other. Do not forget to percuss over the clavicles and on the sides of the chest.

Auscultation of the chest

! Warm the diaphragm of your stethoscope.

○ If old enough, ask the child to take deep breaths through the mouth and, using the diaphragm of the stethoscope, auscultate the chest. Start at the apex of one lung, and compare one side to the other. Are the breath sounds vesicular or bronchial? Are there any added sounds?

After the examination

Ask to look at the sputum pot.

Indicate that you might like to measure the PEFR (see Chapter 16, *Instruct on the use of a PEFR meter*) and, if necessary, order a chest X-ray.

Cover the child.

Thank the child and parent.

Summarise your findings and offer a differential diagnosis.

Most common conditions likely to come up in a *Paediatric examination: respiratory system* OSCE:

▷ Asthma.

▷ Broncho-pulmonary dysplasia.

▷ Cystic fibrosis.

46. Paediatric examination: abdomen

Before starting

Introduce yourself to the child and the parent.

Tell the child that you are going to examine his abdomen.

Position him so that he is lying flat and expose his abdomen as much as possible (customarily "nipples to knees", but this is not appropriate in an OSCE setting).

Ensure that he is comfortable.

The examination

General inspection

- From the end of the couch, observe the child's general appearance:
  - Does the child look his age? (Mention the growth chart).
  - Nutritional status.
  - State of health/other obvious signs.
- Inspect the abdomen noting any:
  - Distension.
  - Localised masses.
  - Scars and skin changes.

! A distended abdomen is often a normal finding in younger infants.

Inspection and examination of the hands

- Take both hands, looking for:
  - Clubbing.
  - Nail signs.

Inspection and examination of the head, neck and upper body

- Inspect the sclera for signs of jaundice or anaemia.
- Inspect the mouth, looking for ulcers (Crohn's disease), angular stomatitis (nutritional deficiency), atrophic glossitis (iron deficiency, vitamin B12 deficiency, folate deficiency), furring of the tongue (loss of appetite) and the state of the dentition.
- Examine the neck for lymphadenopathy.

Palpation of the abdomen

Abdominal palpation can be difficult in children because they do not relax the abdominal muscles. Attempt to distract the child by handing him a toy or try to get him to relax by coaxing him into palpating his abdomen and then copying his actions.

! Ask the child if he has any tummy pain and keep your eyes on the child's face as you palpate his abdomen.

- *Light palpation* – Begin by palpating furthest from the area of pain or discomfort and systematically palpate in the four quadrants and in the umbilical area. Look for tenderness, guarding, and any masses.
- *Deep palpation* – For greater precision. Describe and localise any masses.

Palpation of the organs

- *Liver* – Starting in the right lower quadrant, feel for the liver edge using the flat of your hand. Note that the liver edge can usually be palpated in younger infants.
- *Spleen* – Palpate for the spleen as for the liver, again starting in the right lower quadrant.
- *Kidneys* – Position the child close to the edge of the bed and ballot each kidney using the technique of deep bimanual palpation. Beyond the neonatal period, it is unlikely that you should feel a normal kidney.

Percussion

- Percuss the liver area, also remembering to detect its upper border.
- Percuss the suprapubic area for dullness (bladder distension).
- If the abdomen is distended, test for shifting dullness (ascites).

Auscultation

- Auscultate in the mid-abdomen for abdominal sounds. Listen for 30 seconds before concluding that they are hyperactive, hypoactive or absent.

Examination of the groins and genitals

- This should be mentioned but is usually not performed in an OSCE. Inspect the groins for any hernias and, in boys, examine the testes (this is particularly important in younger infants).

Rectal examination

- This is not common practice in paediatrics and is avoided unless specifically indicated. Mention that you might inspect the anus for fissures.

After examining the patient

Ask to test the urine.

Cover the child.

Thank the child and parent.

Summarise your findings and offer a differential diagnosis.

> **Most common conditions likely to come up in a *Paediatric examination: abdomen* OSCE:**
>
> ▷ Constipation.   ▷ Kidney transplant.
>
> ▷ Coeliac disease.

47. Paediatric examination: gait and neurological function

Examination of neurological function in children is principally a matter of observation. If the child is old enough to obey commands, a more formal assessment of gait and neurological function can be carried out, as for adults.

The examination

Neurological overview

- A brief developmental assessment should be performed to enable you to gauge the child's subsequent performance. Ask the parent the child's age and ask him if he has any concerns about the child's vision and/or hearing.

Gait and movement

- If the child is too young to walk, observe him crawling or playing. Is he using all his limbs equally?
- If this is possible, observe the child walking and running. Common abnormalities of gait in children include:
  - Scissoring or tiptoeing gait – suggestive of cerebral palsy or of Duchenne muscular dystrophy.
  - Broad-based gait – suggestive of a cerebellar disorder.
  - Limp – limps have many causes such as a dislocated hip, trauma, sepsis and arthritis. Is the limp painful or painless?
- If this is possible, observe the child get up from the floor. Gower's sign (the child climbing up his legs) is suggestive of Duchenne's muscular dystrophy.

Inspection

- Inspect all four limbs, in particular looking for muscle wasting or hypertrophy. Hypertrophy of the calves is suggestive of Duchenne's muscular dystrophy.

Tone

- Assess tone and range of movement in all four limbs.
- In younger children also assess truncal tone: can the child sit unsupported?
- Test head lag in young infants.

Power

○ Again observation is key as this is difficult to test in children. Observe the child playing, and look out for appropriate anti-gravity movement.

Reflexes

○ Check all reflexes as in the adult. Practice is the key! Eliciting the Babinski sign (extensor plantar reflex) is not very useful in children.

Co-ordination

○ If the child is old enough to obey commands, assess co-ordination by the finger-to-nose test or just by asking the child to jump or hop. In the child cannot obey commands, give him a toy or some bricks and assess co-ordination by observing him at play.

Sensation

○ Indicate that you would test sensation.

Cranial nerves

○ Indicate that you would test the cranial nerves. If possible, this is done exactly as in the adult.

After examining the child

Thank the parent and child.

Summarise your findings and offer a differential diagnosis.

Most common conditions likely to come up in a _Paediatric examination: gait and neurological function_ OSCE:

○ Cerebral palsy.

○ Ex-premature infant.

○ Duchenne muscular dystrophy.

48. Perform Basic Life Support on an infant or child

Specifications: A mannequin in lieu of an infant or child.

Note: For the purposes of Basic Life Support, an infant is defined as being of less than 1 year of age, and a child is defined as being from ages 1 to 8.

Ensure a safe approach.

Shout, "Are you all right?" *Do not shake.*

If there is no response, shout for help.

Airway

○ Open the child's airway by the head-tilt, chin-lift method. If you are having trouble opening the airway, turn the child onto his back and try again. Avoid doing a head-tilt in cases of suspected neck injury.

○ Remove any visible obstruction from the mouth.

Breathing

○ Holding the child's airway open, put your ear to his mouth. *Listen*, *feel* and *look* for breathing for 10 seconds.

→ If he is breathing normally, place him on his side and find help. Then reassess his breathing.

○ If he is not breathing normally, give two effective rescue breaths, ensuring that the chest rises and falls. The technique for the child is similar to that for the adult. In the infant, you must make your mouth cover both the infant's mouth and nose (the mouth to mouth-and-nose technique). In either case, ensure head tilt and chin lift at all times.

→ If after five attempts, despite having re-checked the mouth and having corrected your head-tilt chin-lift technique, you still cannot deliver two effective rescue breaths, move on to the foreign body airway obstruction sequence.

Circulation

○ In the child, feel for the carotid pulse for 10 seconds. Never feel for both carotid pulses simultaneously. In the infant, feel for the brachial pulse for 10 seconds.

→ If there are signs of circulation (or pulse rate > 60 beats per minute), continue rescue breathing and re-check for circulation every minute.

○ If there are no signs of circulation (or pulse rate < 60 beats per minute) or you are unsure, begin cardiopulmonary resuscitation.

○ If you are alone, you should perform cardiopulmonary resuscitation for 1 minute before calling for help.

○ After having summoned help, continue cardiopulmonary resuscitation until the child makes a movement or takes a spontaneous breath. If this fails to happen, continue until help arrives, or until exhaustion.

Paediatric cardiac massage technique		
	Infant	**Child**
Use	Tips of two fingers	Heel of hand
Position	One finger breadth inferior to nipple line	One finger breadth above xiphisternum
Depth	1/3 of chest	1/3 of chest
Ratio	5:1	5:1
Rate	100 per minute	100 per minute

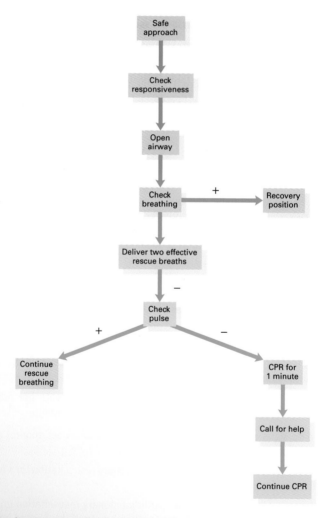

Figure 7. Paediatric Basic Life Support flowchart

49. Child immunisation programme

The UK immunisation schedule		
Age	**Vaccine**	**Specifications**
Birth	BCG	If at risk of tuberculosis
2 months	DTP triple vaccine: ○ diphtheria ○ tetanus ○ pertussis Hib Meningococcus type C Polio	
3 months	As for 2 months	
4 months	As for 2 months	
12–15 months	MMR: ○ measles ○ mumps ○ rubella	
3½ years (pre-school age)	Diphtheria Tetanus Polio MMR	Boosters
10–14 years	BCG	If indicated
16 years (school leavers)	Diphtheria Tetanus Polio	Boosters

The MMR controversy

- Measles can cause fits, encephalitis, pneumonia, sub-acute sclerosing pancencephalitis (SSPE) and death.

- Mumps can cause meningitis, encephalitis, deafness, and sterility.

- Rubella in pregnancy can cause severe damage to the foetus.

- The MMR vaccine is safe and effective, and 500 million doses of the vaccine have been given since 1972.

- Common side-effects of the MMR vaccine are a sore injection site and flu-like symptoms. Very rarely, an allergic reaction can occur.

- No evidence has been found to support a distinct syndrome of MMR-induced autism or inflammatory bowel disease.

- Separate administration of the measles, mumps and rubella vaccines provides no added benefit over administration of the combined MMR vaccine, but on the contrary, could result in delayed or missed vaccinations.

Be prepared for an OSCE station involving a concerned parent, and keep up to date on the latest developments surrounding the issue.

50. Take a geriatric history

Before starting

Introduce yourself to the patient.

Explain that you are going to ask him some questions to determine the nature of his problems, and ask for his consent to do this.

Ensure that he is comfortable; if not, make sure that he is.

Find out if you can take a collateral history from a caretaker.

The history

- Name and age.

Presenting complaint and history of presenting complaint

- Enquire about the presenting complaint.

Ask about:

- Physical independence. Describe a typical day.
- Living arrangements. Housing, stairs, heating, poor lighting, slippery bathtubs, loose rugs, etc.
- Carers and support services.
- Social interaction. Family, friends, clubs, etc.
- Mood. Ask if the patient sleeps OK, enjoys food, sometimes feels sad.
- Daily diet.
- Dizziness.
- Falls.
- Incontinence.
- Mental status. If appropriate, perform an abbreviated mental test.
- Smoking.
- Alcohol consumption.

Past medical history

- Current, past and childhood illnesses. Ask about rheumatic fever and polio.
- Surgery.
- Recent visits to the doctor.

Drug history

- Prescribed medication and *compliance*.
- Over-the-counter drugs.
- Allergies.

Family history

▷ Parents, siblings and children. Ask specifically about Alzheimer's disease, cancer and diabetes.

After taking the history

Ask the patient if there is anything that he might add that you have forgotten to ask.

Thank the patient.

Formulate a problem list.

51. Examine an elderly patient

Examining an elderly patient is very similar to examining a patient of any other age. If asked to examine an elderly patient, important features to look out for or aspects to consider are:

General inspection

Nutritional status, posture, tremor, gait.

Cardiovascular system

Blood pressure (lying and standing), arrhythmias, added sounds, murmurs, ankle oedema, carotid bruits, absent peripheral pulses.

Respiratory system

Respiratory rate, chest expansion, basal crackles (may be difficult to hear due to basilar rales).

Abdomen

Dentition, organomegaly, bladder distension, abdominal aortic aneurysm, frequency and quality of abdominal sounds, rectal examination.

Neurological system

Vision, power, co-ordination.

Musculoskeletal system

Arthritis, muscle wasting, contractures.

Skin

Pressure sores, senile keratosis, senile purpura, bruises, pre-malignant or malignant lesions.

52. Take a dermatological history

Before starting

Introduce yourself to the patient.

Explain that you are going to ask him some questions to uncover the nature of his skin problem, and ask for his consent to do this.

Ensure that he is comfortable; if not, make sure that he is.

The history

○ Name and age.

Presenting complaint

○ Ask the patient to describe his skin problem.

History of presenting complaint

Ask about:

○ When, where and how the problem started.

○ What the initial lesions looked like and how they have evolved.

○ Symptoms: especially pain, pruritus and bleeding.

○ Aggravating factors such as sunlight, heat, soaps, etc.

Past medical history

○ Previous skin disease.

○ Atopic symptoms (allergic rhinitis, asthma, childhood eczema).

○ Past or present medical illnesses.

○ Surgery.

Drug history

○ Prescribed and self-administered medicaments, including creams (present and previous).

○ Cosmetics and moisturising creams (present and previous).

○ Allergies.

Family history

○ Medical history of parents, siblings and children, focusing on skin problems.

○ Sexual contacts.

Social history

- Occupation (in detail). Does the skin problem improve when on holiday?
- Hobbies (in detail).
- Home background.
- Alcohol consumption.
- Travel, especially to the tropics.

Systems review

(If appropriate).

After taking the history

Ask the patient if there is anything that he might add that you have forgotten to ask.

Thank the patient.

Summarise your findings and offer a differential diagnosis.

53. Examine the skin

Introduce yourself to the patient.

Explain the examination and ask for his consent to carry it out.

Ask him to undress to his undergarments.

Ensure that he is comfortable.

Ask him to report any pain or discomfort during the examination.

Ensure adequate lighting.

The examination

- Describe the distribution and colour of the lesion(s). Look at all parts of the body.

- Describe the morphology of the individual lesions, commenting on their size, shape, borders, elevation and spatial relationship. Use precise dermatological terms.

- Note any secondary skin lesions such as scaling, lichenification, crusting, excoriation, erosion, ulceration, and scarring.

- Palpate the lesions. Assess their consistency. Do they blanch?

- Examine the nails.

- Examine the hair.

- Examine the mucous membranes.

- Check for lymphadenopathy, if appropriate.

- Check the pedal pulses, if appropriate.

After the examination

Offer to help the patient put his clothes back on.

Thank the patient.

Wash your hands.

Summarise your findings and offer a differential diagnosis.

Most common conditions likely to come up in an *Examine the skin* OSCE:

- Psoriasis.
- Eczema.
- Contact dermatitis.
- Acne vulgaris.
- Erythema nodosum.

54. Give advice on sun protection

! **Also see Chapter 85, *Explaining skills*.**

Before starting

Introduce yourself to the patient.

Tell him what you are going to explain, and determine how much he already knows.

The advice

Explain that there are three types of ultra violet radiation from the sun: UVA, UVB and UVC.

▷ UVA and UVB can cause skin cancer.

▷ UVC does not reach the surface of the earth and is therefore of no concern.

Explain that, other than causing skin cancer, UV radiation can also cause the skin to burn and (horror!) to age prematurely.

UV levels depend on a number of factors such as time of day, time of year, latitude, altitude, cloud cover and ozone covering.

Explain that there are four methods of protecting oneself against the sun's rays:

1. Avoiding the outdoors. The UVA and UVB rays are most direct around midday and one should therefore avoid being outside from 11 am to 2 pm.

2. Seeking shade.

3. Covering up (including a hat and sunglasses that conform to British standard 2724).

4. Applying sunscreen.

▷ A sunscreen's star rating is a measure of its level of protection against UVA.

▷ A sunscreen's Sun Protection Factor (SPF) is a measure of its level of protection against UVB.

▷ It is advisable to use a sunscreen that has a star rating of at least three stars *** and an SPF of at least 15.

▷ Sunscreen should be applied thickly over all sun-exposed areas.

▷ Sunscreen should be re-applied regularly.

! **Sunscreens should not be used as a means to spend more time in the sun.**

Finally, advise the patient to report any moles that change in colour, shape, texture or size.

After giving the advice

Summarise the information and ensure that the patient has understood it.

Ask the patient if he has any questions or concerns.

Give the patient a leaflet on sun protection.

55. Take an obstetric history

Specifications: You might be asked to concentrate on only certain aspects of the obstetric history.

Before starting

Introduce yourself to the patient.

Explain that you are going to ask her some questions to uncover the nature and background of her obstetric complaint, and ask for her consent to do this.

Ensure that she is comfortable.

The history

- Name, age and occupation.
- Is the pregnancy planned or unplanned? If it is unplanned, is it *desired*?

History of previous pregnancies (past reproductive history)

For each previous pregnancy, ask about:

The pregnancy:

- The date (year).
- The duration.
- The mode of delivery.
- The outcome.

The child:

- The child's birth-weight.
- The child's present condition.

! **Do not forget to ask about terminations and miscarriages.**

History of present pregnancy

- Determine the duration of gestation and calculate the expected due date (EDD):
  - Ask about the date of the patient's last menstrual period (LMP).
  - Ask if her periods had been regular prior to her LMP.
  - Ask if she had been on the oral contraceptive pill (OCP). If she had been on the OCP, determine when she stopped taking it and the number of menses she had before becoming pregnant.
  - Determine the duration of gestation and calculate the EDD. To calculate the EDD add 9 months and 7 days to the date of the LMP. Alternatively, add one year, subtract 3 months, and add 7 days.

▷ Ask about foetal movements and about any change in their frequency.

▷ Take a detailed history of the pregnancy, enquiring about:

First trimester:

▷ Date and method of pregnancy confirmation.

▷ Symptoms of pregnancy.

▷ Ultrasound scan.

▷ Chorionic villus sampling.

▷ Type of antenatal care.

Second trimester:

▷ Amniocentesis.

▷ Anomaly scan.

▷ Quickening.

Third trimester:

▷ Findings at antenatal clinic. You *must* ask about blood pressure and proteinuria.

▷ Vaginal bleeding.

▷ Hospital admissions.

Presenting problem (presenting complaint)

Ask about the presenting symptoms in detail.

Gynaecological history

Take a relevant gynaecological history, and ask about the date and result of the last cervical smear test.

Past medical history

▷ Current, past and childhood illnesses.

▷ Surgery.

▷ Recent visits to the doctor.

Drug history

▷ Prescribed medication.

▷ Over-the-counter drugs.

▷ Illicit drugs.

▷ Allergies.

Family history

- Parents, siblings, children. Has anyone in the family had a similar problem?

Social history

- Employment.
- Income and financial support.
- Housing and family living at home.
- Smoking.
- Alcohol intake.

After taking the history

Ask the patient if there is anything she might add that you have forgotten to ask about.

Thank the patient.

If asked, summarise your findings and offer a differential diagnosis.

56. Examine the pregnant woman

Specifications: Often an anatomical model in lieu of a patient.

Before examining the patient

Introduce yourself to the patient.

Explain the examination and ensure consent.

Indicate that you would weigh the patient, take her blood pressure (pre-eclampsia), test her urine (pre-eclampsia, gestational diabetes) and ask her to empty her bladder.

Position the patient.

Expose her abdomen.

Ensure that she is comfortable.

The examination

Inspection

- Abdominal distension and symmetry.
- Foetal movements.
- *Linea nigra.*
- *Striae gravidarum.*
- Scars.

Palpation of the abdomen

Determine the:

- Size of the uterus.
- Number of foetuses.
- Size of the foetus(es).
- Lie.
- Presenting part.
- Engagement.

Some important definitions

- **Lie.** The relationship of the long axis of the foetus to that of the uterus, described as longitudinal, transverse or oblique.

- **Presenting part.** The part of the foetus that is in relation with the pelvic inlet.

- **Engagement.** Described in fifths of head palpable above the pelvic inlet.

Symphyseal–fundal height (SFH)

Using a tape measure, measure from the mid-point of the symphysis pubis to the top of the uterus. From 20 to 38 weeks of gestation, the SFH in centimetres approximates to the number of weeks of gestation.

Auscultation

Listen to the foetal heart by placing a pinard stethoscope over the foetus' anterior shoulder.

After the examination

Cover the patient up.

Thank the patient.

Summarise your findings.

57. Take a gynaecological history

Specifications: You might be asked to concentrate on only certain aspects of the gynaecological history.

Before starting

Introduce yourself to the patient.

Explain that you are going to ask her some questions to uncover the nature and background of her gynaecological complaint, and ask for her consent to do this.

Ensure that she is comfortable.

The history

○ Name, age and occupation.

Presenting complaint and history of presenting complaint

○ Enquire in detail about the nature of the presenting complaint and the history of the presenting complaint. First listen to the patient. Then ask about:

- ○ Age at menarche.
- ○ Regularity of menses.
- ○ Dysmenorrhoea.
- ○ Date of LMP. Did the LMP seem normal?
- ○ Vaginal discharge. If there is a vaginal discharge, ask about its amount, colour and smell. Is it causing any itching?
- ○ Date and result of last cervical smear test.
- ○ Vaginal prolapse.
- ○ Urinary incontinence.
- ○ Coitus, present or past. ("Are you sexually active?").
- ○ Dyspareunia.
- ○ Use of contraception.

Past medical history

○ Past gynaecological history.

○ Past reproductive history: previous pregnancies in chronological order, including terminations and miscarriages.

○ Past medical history.

- ○ Current, past and childhood illnesses.
- ○ Surgery.
- ○ Recent visits to the doctor.

Drug history

- Prescribed medication.
- Over-the-counter drugs.
- Illicit drugs.
- Allergies.

Family history

- Ask about parents, siblings, children. Has anyone in the family had a similar problem? In the case of a suspected STD, don't forget to ask about the partner.

Social history

- Employment.
- Housing and home-help.
- Travel.
- Smoking.
- Alcohol consumption.

After taking the history

Ask the patient if there is anything she might add that you have forgotten to ask about.

Thank the patient.

If asked, summarise your findings and offer a differential diagnosis.

58. Perform a gynaecological (bimanual) examination

Specifications: A pelvic model in lieu of a patient.

Before starting

Introduce yourself to the patient.

Explain the examination, reassuring the patient that although it may be a bit uncomfortable, it should not be painful.

Obtain consent.

If you are male, ask for a female chaperone.

Confirm that the patient has emptied her bladder.

Indicate that you would carry out an abdominal examination prior to the gynaecological examination.

Once undressed, ask the patient to lie flat on the couch, bring her heels to her buttocks, and let her knees flop out.

Ensure that she is comfortable, using a drape to cover her up.

The examination

! **Always tell the patient what you are about to do.**

- Don a pair of non-sterile gloves.
- Inspect the vulva, paying close attention to:
  - The pattern of hair distribution.
  - The labia majora.
  - The clitoris.
- Palpate the labia majora.
- Palpate for Bartholin's gland. (This structure is not normally palpable.)

- Lubricate your right glove.
- Use the thumb and index finger of your left hand to separate the labia minora.
- Insert the index and middle fingers of your right hand into the vagina at an angle of 45 degrees.
- Palpate the vaginal walls.
- Use your fingertips to palpate the cervix. Assess the cervix for size, shape, consistency and mobility. Is the cervix tender?
- Palpate the uterus: place the palmar surface of your left hand about 5 cm above the symphysis pubis and the internal fingers of your right hand on the cervix and gently appose your fingers in an attempt to "catch" the uterus. Assess the uterus for size, consistency, and mobility. Can you feel any masses?

- Palpate the right adnexae: place the palmar surface of your left hand in the right iliac fossa and the internal fingers of your right hand in the right fornix and gently appose your fingers in an attempt to "catch" the ovary. Is there any excitation tenderness? (Look at the patient's face).

- Use a similar technique for palpating the left adnexae.

- Once you have removed your internal fingers, inspect the glove for any blood or discharge.

After the examination

Indicate that you could also have carried out a speculum examination and taken a cervical smear (see Chapter 59, *Perform a surgical smear test*).

Give the patient an opportunity to re-dress.

Thank the patient.

Summarise your findings and offer a differential diagnosis.

Most common conditions likely to come up in a *Perform a gynaecological (bimanual) examination* OSCE:

- Uterine fibroids.
- Ovarian cyst.

59. Perform a cervical smear test

Specifications: An anatomical model in lieu of a patient.

Before starting

Introduce yourself to the patient.

Explain the procedure to her, and ask for her consent to carry it out.

Request a chaperone, if appropriate.

Once undressed, ask the patient to lie flat on the couch, to bring her heels to her buttocks, and to let her knees flop out.

Ensure that she is comfortable.

The equipment

On a trolley, gather:

- A pair of gloves.
- An Ayres spatula.
- Fixative spray (or 95% alcohol).
- A bivalve speculum.
- A brush, if post-menopausal.
- Labelled slides (name, date of birth, hospital number).

The procedure

- Put on gloves.
- Warm the speculum's blades under a stream of tepid water (the water also lubricates the blades).
- Insert the speculum with the screw facing sideways, rotating it into position (screw upwards) and then opening it.
- Adjust the light source to ensure maximum visibility of the vagina.
- Inspect the cervix and identify the transformation zone.

! A smear should not be taken if there is any bleeding or vaginal discharge.

- Place the tip of the Ayres spatula in the external os and rotate the spatula by 360 degrees, keeping it firmly applied to the cervix.
- Spread the material obtained on the spatula evenly onto the slides.
- Immediately spray fixative onto the slides.
- Carefully remove the speculum.

After the procedure

Dispose of the speculum and of the gloves.

Ask the patient if she has any questions or concerns.

Thank the patient.

60. Take a breast history

Introduce yourself to the patient.

Explain that you are going to ask her some questions to uncover the nature of her complaint, and ask for her consent to do this.

Ensure that she is comfortable; if not, make sure that she is.

The history

○ Name, age and occupation. Is the patient pregnant or lactating?

Presenting complaint and history of presenting complaint

○ Ask about the nature of the presenting complaint. Use open questions.

○ Ask specifically about pain, a lump in the breast and nipple discharge.

For pain, determine:

- ○ Nature.
- ○ Site.
- ○ Onset.
- ○ Duration.
- ○ Aggravating and alleviating factors.
- ○ Associated symptoms.
- ○ Cyclicity.
- ○ If the patient has had it before.

For a lump in the breast, determine:

- ○ Onset.
- ○ Duration.
- ○ Cyclicity.
- ○ If it is painful.
- ○ Associated symptoms.
- ○ If the patient has had it before.

For a nipple discharge, determine:

- ○ Amount.
- ○ Colour.
- ○ If it is bilateral.
- ○ If it is from one duct or several.
- ○ If it is spontaneous.
- ○ Associated symptoms.
- ○ If the patient has had it before.

Past medical history

- Current, past, and childhood illnesses.
- Surgery.
- Recent visits to the doctor.

Drug history

- Prescribed medication, especially oral contraceptives and HRT.
- Over-the-counter drugs.
- Illicit drugs.
- Allergies.

Family history

- Parents, siblings and children. Ask specifically about breast problems.

Social history

- Smoking.
- Alcohol consumption.
- Employment, past and present.
- Housing.
- Hobbies.

Systems enquiry

(If appropriate).

After taking the history

Ask the patient if there is anything that she might add that you have forgotten to ask.

Thank the patient.

Summarise your findings and offer a differential diagnosis.

Say that you would like to examine the patient and order some investigations (e.g., mammogram, ultrasound scan, fine-needle aspiration cytology) to confirm your diagnosis.

Most common conditions likely to come up in a *Take a breast history* OSCE:

- Fibroadenoma.
- Fibrocystic disease.
- Mastitis.
- Breast abscess.

- Mammary duct ectasia.
- Carcinoma.
- Intraductal papilloma.

61. Examine the breasts

A complete breast examination involves inspection, palpation of the breast tissue, palpation of the nipple and palpation of the lymph nodes.

Before examining the patient

Introduce yourself to the patient.

Explain the examination to her, and ask for her consent to carry it out.

Request a chaperone, if appropriate.

Ask her to undress from the waist upwards and hand her a blanket to cover herself up.

Ask her to sit on the edge of the couch, and ensure that she is comfortable.

The examination

General inspection

○ From a distance, observe the patient's general appearance (age, state of health).

Inspection of the breasts

○ Note the size, symmetry, contour, and colour of the breast; also note the pattern of venous drainage. In particular, look for the important signs of nipple inversion (or retraction) and *peau d' orange* (breast carcinoma). Also remember to look under the breasts.

○ Now ask the patient to put her hands on her head and then to press them against her hips. Look for tethering and for asymmetrical changes in breast contour.

Palpation of the breasts

○ Ask the patient to sit back on the couch, reclining at 45 degrees.

○ Warm up your hands.

○ Before palpating the breasts, ask if there is any breast or chest pain.

○ Starting with the normal breast, palpate the breast tissue with the palmar surface of the middle three fingers, using an even rotary movement to compress the breast tissue gently towards the chest wall. If the breasts are large, use one hand to steady the breast on its lower border.

○ Examine each breast following a concentric trail.

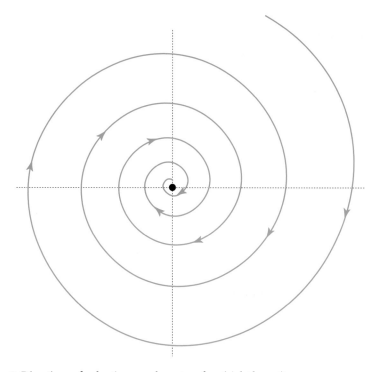

Figure 8. Directions of palpation over breast surface (right breast)

- Ask the patient to rest her arms above her head and palpate the tail of Spence between thumb and forefinger.

! Remember that there are two breasts.

Palpation of the nipple

- Hold the nipple between thumb and forefinger and gently compress it, in an attempt to express a discharge (a discharge could mean duct ectasia, a carcinoma or an intraductal papilloma). Any fluid expressed should be smeared for cytology and swabbed for microbiology.

Palpation of the lymph nodes

- Expose the right axilla by lifting and abducting the arm and supporting it at the wrist with your right hand.
- With the left hand, palpate the following lymph node groups:
  - the apical
  - the anterior

- the posterior
- the infraclavicular and supraclavicular
- the nodes on the medial aspect of the humerus.
- Now expose the left axilla by lifting and abducting the left arm and supporting it at the wrist with your left hand.
- With your right hand, palpate the lymph node groups, as listed above.

! Assess any nodes for size, shape, consistency, mobility and tenderness.

After examining the breasts

Cover the patient up.

Thank the patient.

Summarise your findings and offer a differential diagnosis.

> **Most common conditions likely to come up in an *Examine the breasts* OSCE:**
>
> - Fibroadenoma.
> - Fibrocystic disease.
> - Carcinoma (unlikely to come up but you might be asked about it).

62. Explain the use of pessaries and suppositories

This section provides just the facts. For the communications skills involved, refer to Chapter 85, *Explaining skills*.

What they are

Like tablets, they are medication.

- Suppositories are for rectal use, examples being pain-killers and steroids.
- Pessaries are for vaginal use, examples being antibiotics and progesterone.

! **To confuse matters, some preparations can be used via either route.**

Why they are used

They are used if:

- Oral drugs cannot be given, for example, in the post-operative period or if the patient is vomiting.
- The site of action of the drug is the rectum or vagina, or near enough, for example, the cervix.

How they are used

Because they liquefy at room temperature, pessaries and suppositories should be stored in a cool place, and should only be removed from their packaging prior to insertion.

Suppositories should be inserted through the anus into the rectum to a depth of about 2–3 cm, using a finger.

Pessaries should be placed, using a gloved finger, as high into the vagina as possible.

! **Be sensitive to the cultural and social issues involved in placing a finger into the vagina or rectum, and be sympathetic and understanding.**

After they are used

Advocate thorough hand ablutions. The patient should then lie still.

63. Take a sexual history

! This is a history that students usually find difficult because of the highly personal nature of the questions that must be asked. The secret is to remain formal and professional throughout.

Before starting

Introduce yourself to the patient.

Set the scene: "I'd like to ask you a few questions about your sex life. I don't mean to embarrass you, and it's all right if you prefer not to answer some of my questions. May I begin?"

Reassure the patient about confidentiality, if necessary.

The history

Who

- Who did you last have sex with, and when was this?
- Who else have you had sex with in the past three months?
- Were they regular or casual partners?
- Were they male or female (or both)?

How

- Did you have vaginal/oral/anal sex?
- If oral or anal sex, did you give it or receive it?
- Did you use protection on each occasion?
- If yes, did you use it successfully?
- Have you ever been hurt or abused by your partner?

Where

- Have you had sex abroad?
- Where are your partners from?
- Is it possible that they have had sex abroad?

Sexually transmitted diseases

Ask about:

- Any sores, discharge, itching, dysuria and abdominal pain (in females). Explore any symptoms.
- History of sexually transmitted diseases (including HIV) in both the patient and his partner(s).
- In females, date and result of the last cervical smear test.

Sexual function

▷ Do you have any problems with, or concerns about, having sex?

Past medical history

Drug history and allergies

Family history

Social history

After taking the history

Ask if there is anything the patient would like to add which you might have forgotten to ask about.

Thank the patient.

Summarise your findings and suggest a further course of action.

64. Perform an HIV risk assessment

Before starting

Introduce yourself to the patient.

Explain that you are going to ask him some questions to determine the likelihood of his having contracted HIV, and ask him for his consent to do this.

Remember to be especially sensitive, tactful and empathic.

HIV risk assessment

○ Explore the patient's reason for attendance.

Sex

Establish:

○ If the patient has sex with men, women or both.

○ If he has had unprotected anal, vaginal, or oral sex. If so, when, where, how often and with how many different partners? Receptive anal intercourse is especially high risk.

○ If he has recently contracted any sexually transmitted diseases.

○ The HIV status and sexual practices of the patient's partner(s).

Illicit intravenous drug use

Establish:

○ If the patient has been injecting himself. If so, has he shared needles?

○ If any of his partners inject themselves.

Blood products and transfusions

Establish:

○ If the patient is haemophiliac.

○ If he has received blood products or transfusions prior to about 1985.

○ If any of his partners are haemophiliac or have received blood products or transfusions prior to about 1985.

○ Ask about the patient's occupation to determine if he poses a professional risk.

Before finishing

Ask the patient if there is anything he might add that you have forgotten to ask about.

Give him feedback on his HIV risk, and indicate a further course of action if appropriate.

Address his anxieties.

Thank the patient.

65. Explain the use of a condom

Introduce yourself to the patient.

Establish how much he already knows about using condoms.

The equipment

- Two condoms.
- A model of a penis.
- An information booklet on condoms.

Explaining the use of a condom

Explain that condom use should be discussed with the partner(s) and that the condom should be put on before any genital contact.

Demonstrate to:

- Check for the British Kite mark (a guarantee of quality).
- Check that the expiry date has not passed.
- Carefully tear open the pack and remove the condom.
- Position the condom on the tip of the erect penis.
- Squeeze out the air from the tip of the condom and gently roll it out to the base of the penis.
- Hold the condom at the base of the penis during penetration.
- Remove the condom ensuring that semen is not spilt.
- Dispose of the condom in the bin (condoms must never be re-used).

Ask the patient to repeat the procedure.

! Explain to the patient that condoms can occasionally tear and that, in this event, he and his partner should consult a GP or family planning clinic.

After explaining the use of a condom

Ask if the patient has any questions or concerns.

Tell him to come back if he should have any further questions.

Give him the information booklet on condoms.

66. Prescribe the combined oral contraceptive pill

Before starting

Introduce yourself to the patient.

Ask for her name and age.

Confirm her reason for attendance.

Has she considered other methods of contraception? If the pill remains her method of choice, go through:

Prescribing the contraceptive pill: items to cover

Efficacy

- 99.9% if used correctly; 97% in practice. Does not protect against STDs.

Principal benefits

- Periods – more regular, less blood loss, fewer period pains.
- Cancers – decreased risk of ovarian cancer and of endometrial cancer.
- Acne – often improves.

Principal risks

- Clotting – increased risk of deep venous thrombosis and of pulmonary embolism.
- Cardiovascular – increased risk of myocardial infarction.
- Cancers – increased risk of breast cancer and of adenoma of the cervix.

Principal adverse effects

- Headache
- Nausea
- Dizziness
- Hypertension
- Breast tenderness
- Weight gain
- Depression

Principal contraindications

ABSOLUTE

- Thrombophlebitis, thromboembolitic disorder or history of thromboembolism.
- Stroke.
- Ischaemic heart disease.

- Kidney failure.
- Liver disease.
- History of breast cancer or other oestrogen-dependent cancer of the reproductive organs.
- Pregnancy.

RELATIVE

- Uncontrolled hypertension.
- Migraine.
- Smoking ($>$ 15 cigarettes per day and over the age of 35).
- Abnormal vaginal bleeding.
- Sickle cell disease.
- Breast feeding.
- History or family history of hyperlipidaemia, heart disease or kidney disease.

! Remember to take a drug history, as many common drugs such as ampicillin or carbamazepine can alter the effectiveness of the pill.

Taking the pills

- Start taking pills on the first Sunday after periods begin.
- Take one pill a day at the same time every day for either 21 or 28 days, depending on the number of pills in the pack.
  - After finishing the 28-day pack, start another one immediately. (The last seven pills in the 28-day pack are "dummy pills").
  - After finishing the 21-day pack, stop taking the pill for 7 days. Then start another pack.
- Use barrier contraception for in the first month on the pill.
- If you have vomiting or diarrhoea, use barrier contraception until your next period.

Missing pills

If one pill is missed...

- Take the pill as soon as you remember.
- Take the next pill at the regular time.
- Use barrier contraception for 7 days.

If two pills are missed...

▶ Take two pills a day for 2 days.

▶ Use barrier contraception for 7 days.

If three pills are missed...

▶ Stop taking the pill and start another pack in 7 days time.

Finally

Summarise and check understanding.

Instruct the patient to report any severe or unexpected symptoms.

67. Perform the GALS screening examination

GALS: "Gait, arms, legs and spine". Remember that GALS is a screening test, and that detailed examination is therefore not called for.

Before starting

Introduce yourself to the patient.

Explain the examination and ask for his consent to carry it out.

Ask him to undress to his undergarments.

Ensure that he is comfortable.

The GALS examination

Short history

- Name, age and occupation.
- Do you have any pain or stiffness in your muscles, back, or joints?
- Do you have any difficulty in climbing stairs?
- Do you have any difficulty dressing or washing yourself?

The examination

General inspection

Observe the patient standing. Note any obvious scars, swellings, deformities, or unusual posturing.

Spine

LOOK

- From the front.
- From behind, looking in particular for lumbar lordosis and scoliosis.
- From the side, looking in particular for kyphosis and fixed flexion deformity.

FEEL

- Press on each vertebral body in turn, trying to elicit tenderness.

MOVE

- Bend to touch toes. Look for loss of lumbar lordosis, scoliosis (it often becomes more pronounced) and normal range of movement.

Ask the patient to sit down on the couch.

- Lateral flexion of neck. Put ear on shoulder.
- Flexion and extension of neck. Put chin on chest.
- Spinal rotation. Rotate upper body to either side.

Arms

LOOK

- ▷ Skin: Rashes, nodules, nail signs.
- ▷ Muscles: Wasting, fasciculation.
- ▷ Joints: Asymmetry, swelling, and deformity.

! **Don't forget to inspect both surfaces of the hand.**

FEEL

- ▷ Skin: Temperature.
- ▷ Muscles: General muscle bulk.
- ▷ Joints: Tenderness and warmth. Squeeze each hand at the level of the carpal and metacarpal joints, and try to localise any tenderness by squeezing each individual joint in turn.

MOVE

Ask the patient to copy your movements. Is there any pain or restricted range of movement?

- ▷ Hands: 1. Power grip. Test the strength of the grip by asking the patient to squeeze your finger.

  2. Precision pinch grip. Test the strength of the grip by trying to "break" the pinch.
- ▷ Wrists: Flexion and extension.
- ▷ Elbows: Flexion and extension.
- ▷ Shoulders: Full external rotation and abduction (hands behind head).

Legs

Ask the patient to lie on the couch.

LOOK

- ▷ Skin: Rashes, nodules, callosities on the soles of the feet.
- ▷ Muscles: Wasting, fasciculation.
- ▷ Joints: Asymmetry, swelling and deformity.

FEEL

- ▷ Skin: Temperature.
- ▷ Joints: Tenderness, warmth and swelling. Palpate each knee along the joint margin. Squeeze each foot, and try to localise any tenderness by squeezing each individual joint in turn.

MOVE

- ▷ Bend each knee up in turn.
- ▷ Hold the knee and hip at 90 degrees of flexion and internally rotate the hip. Keep an eye on the patient's face as this is done.
- ▷ Next, put one hand on the knee joint and extend it, feeling for any crepitus.

Gait

Ask the patient to walk, observing:

- ▷ General features: rhythm, speed, limp.
- ▷ The phases of gait: heel-strike, stance, push-off and swing.
- ▷ Transfer ability: sitting and standing from a chair (this should already have been observed).

After completing the examination

Thank the patient.

Offer to help dressing the patient.

Ensure that he is comfortable.

Summarise your findings.

68. Take a rheumatological history

Before starting

Introduce yourself to the patient.

Explain that you are going to ask him some questions to uncover the nature of his complaint, and ask him for his consent to do this.

Ensure that he is comfortable.

The history

○ Name, age and occupation.

Presenting complaint

○ Pain: Ask about any pain and determine its site (i.e., which joints), characteristics and timing. Is there any swelling?

○ Stiffness: Ask about difficulty in starting or carrying out movement.

History of presenting complaint

Ask about:

○ The circumstances of disease onset.

○ The subsequent course of the disease.

○ Any associated features:

   ○ Local: e.g., Inflammation, deformity, cracking, clicking, locking, loss of movement.

   ○ Systemic: e.g., Skin problems, eye problems, GI disturbances.

   ○ General: e.g., Malaise, fever, loss of weight.

○ Possible trauma or infection.

Social history

Ask the patient:

○ If he has any difficulty in doing things, and about the effect that this has on his life.

○ To describe a typical day: getting out of bed, toileting, dressing, etc.

○ About housing and home-help.

○ About mood, and about some of the key features of depression such as sleep disturbance, lethargy, anhedonia.

○ The one thing that he would like to do that he cannot at present.

And, as in any history, don't forget to ask about:

- Travel.
- Smoking.
- Alcohol intake.

Past medical history

- Current, past and childhood illnesses.
- Surgery.
- Recent visits to the doctor.

Drug history

- Prescribed medication, e.g., NSAIDs, steroids, immunosuppressants.
- Over-the-counter drugs.
- Illicit drugs.
- Allergies.

Family history

- Parents, siblings, children. Has anyone in the family had a similar problem?

After taking the history

Ask the patient if there is anything he might add that you have forgotten to ask about.

Thank the patient.

> **Most common conditions likely to come up in a *Take a rheumatological history* OSCE:**
>
> - Rheumatoid arthritis.
> - Osteoarthritis.
> - Psoriatic arthritis.
> - Gout or pseudo-gout.
> - Ankylosing spondylitis.
> - Septic athritis.
> - Polymyositis or dermatomyositis.
> - Polymyalgia rheumatica.
> - Tendon rupture.
> - Complications of steroid treatment.

69. Examine the hand and wrist

Before starting

Introduce yourself to the patient.

Explain the examination and ask for his consent to carry it out.

Ask him to expose his arms.

Ensure that he is comfortable.

The examination

LOOK

First look at the dorsum and then at the palmar surface of the hands.

- Skin: colour, rheumatoid nodules, scars, nail changes.
- Joints: swelling, Heberden's nodes, Bouchard's nodes.
- Shape and position: normal positioning of the hand, ulnar deviation, boutonnière and swan neck deformity of the fingers, finger droop, Z-deformity of the thumb, muscle wasting, Duputyren's contracture.

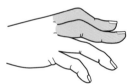

Boutonniere deformity

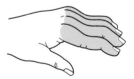

Swan neck deformity

Figure 9. The arthritic hand

FEEL

- Skin: temperature.
- Joints: Swelling, synovial thickening, tenderness.
- Anatomical snuff box (fractured scaphoid).
- Tip of radial styloid and head of ulna.

MOVE

Look for limitation of the normal range of movement, and ask the patient to report any pain.

Wrist

- Flexion and extension.
- Ulnar and radial deviation.
- Pronation and supination.

Thumb

- Extension: stick thumb out to side.
- Abduction: point thumb up to ceiling.
- Adduction: put thumb in palm.
- Opposition: appose thumb to tip of little finger.

Fingers

Each finger should be fully extended and flexed, looking at movements of the metacarpophalangeal and interphalangeal joints. Test the grip strength by asking the patient to squeeze your hand.

Special tests

- Carpal tunnel tests:
    - Try to elicit Tinnel's sign by extending the hand and tapping on the median nerve in the carpal tunnel.
    - Try to elicit Phalen's sign by holding the hand in forceful flexion for at least 30 seconds.
- Flexor profundus: hold a finger extended at the proximal interphalangeal joint and ask the patient to flex the distal interphalangeal joint of that same finger.
- Flexor superficialis: hold all other fingers extended and ask the patient to flex a finger.
- Assess function by asking the patient to use an everyday object such as a pen or a cup.

After the examination

Ask to examine the vascular and neurological systems of the upper limb.

Thank the patient.

Offer to help the patient put his clothes back on.

Offer a differential diagnosis.

Most common conditions likely to come up in an *Examine the hand and wrist* OSCE:

- Osteoarthritis.

- Rheumatoid arthritis.

- Psoriatic arthritis – look at the nails!

- Lesions of the median, radial or ulnar nerves.

- Gout.

- Duputyren's disease.

- De Quervain's tenosynovitis.

- Trigger finger.

70. Examine the elbow

Before starting

Introduce yourself to the patient.

Explain the examination and ask for his consent to carry it out.

Ask him to expose his arms.

Ensure that he is comfortable.

The examination

LOOK

- Overall impression: Varus or valgus deformities (look from behind), effusions, inflammation of the olecranon bursa.
- Skin: Rheumatoid nodules, gouty tophi, scars.
- Muscle wasting: Biceps, triceps, forearm.

FEEL

- Skin: Temperature, rheumatoid nodules, gouty tophi.
- Joints: Tenderness, effusions, synovial thickening.
- Bones: Tenderness of the lateral and medial epicondyles.

MOVE

- Flexion and extension.
- Pronation and suppination.

After examining the elbow

Ask to examine the wrist and hand.

Ask to examine the vascular and neurological systems of the upper limb.

Thank the patient.

Offer to help him put his clothes back on.

Ensure that he is comfortable.

Offer a differential diagnosis.

Most common conditions likely to come up in an *Examine the elbow* OSCE:

- Osteoarthritis.
- Rheumatoid arthritis.
- Olecranon bursitis.

71. Examine the shoulder

Before starting

Introduce yourself to the patient.

Explain the examination and ask for his consent to carry it out.

Ask him to undress from the waist upwards.

Ensure that he is comfortable.

The examination

LOOK

- Overall impression: Alignment, position of arms, axillae, prominence of acromioclavicular and sternoclavicular joints.

- Skin: Colour, sinuses, scars.

- Muscle wasting: Deltoid, periscapular muscles (supra- and infra-spinatus).

FEEL

- Skin: Temperature.

- Bones and joints: Palpate bony landmarks of the shoulder, starting at the sternoclavicular joint and moving out along the clavicle. Try to localise any tenderness. Can you feel any effusions?

- Biceps tendon.

MOVE

Ask the patient to copy your movements, and look for limited range of movement.

- Abduction: Raise arms above head, making the palms of the hands touch.

- Adduction: Move arm across front of body.

- Flexion: Raise arms forwards.

- Extension: Pull arms backwards.

- External rotation: Hold hands behind neck.

- Internal rotation: Reach up back and touch scapulae.

If any one movement is limited, test the passive range of movement.

Serratus anterior function

Ask the patient to put his hands against a wall and to push on it. Observe the scapulae from behind, looking for asymmetry or winging.

After examining the shoulder

Ask to examine the vascular and neurological systems of the upper limb and to examine the neck.

Thank the patient.

Offer to help him put his clothes back on.

Ensure that he is comfortable.

Offer a differential diagnosis.

 Most common conditions likely to come up in an *Examine the shoulder* OSCE:

- Frozen shoulder.
- Acute calcific tendonitis.
- Rotator cuff tear.
- Winging of the scapula.
- Bicipital tendonitis.

- Osteoarthritis.
- Referred pain from cervical spine or from the heart.
- Rupture of long head of biceps (*Popeye's sign*).

72. Examine the spine

Before starting

Introduce yourself to the patient.

Explain the examination and ask for his consent to carry it out.

Ask him to undress to his undergarments.

Ensure that he is comfortable.

The examination

LOOK

- General inspection: ask the patient to stand and assess his posture. Are there any obvious malformations?
- Skin: scars, pigmentation, abnormal hair, unusual skin creases.
- Shape and posture:
  - Spine:
    - Lateral deviation of the spine – a *list*.   (Observe from the back)
    - Lateral curvature of the spine – *scoliosis*.   (Observe from the back)
    - Too much bending of the spine – *kyphosis*. (Observe from the side)
    - Bending of the spine on a hinge – a *kyphos*. (Observe from the side)
    - Loss of lumbar lordosis.
  - Asymmetry or malformation of the chest.
  - Asymmetry of the pelvis.

FEEL

- Palpate and percuss the spinous processes and interspinous ligaments.

MOVE

Ask the patient to copy your movements, looking for any limitation of range of movement. Ask the patient to indicate if any of the movements are painful.

Gait

Neck

- Flexion.
- Extension.
- Lateral flexion.

Thoracic spine

▷ Rotation. (Ask patient to sit or stabilise his pelvis.)

Measure chest expansion. It should be at least 5 cm.

Lumbar spine

▷ Flexion (touch toes).

▷ Extension (lean back).

▷ Lateral flexion (slide hand alongside leg).

Measure the lumbar excursion.

Special tests

Ask the patient to lie prone.

▷ Palpate the sacroiliac joints.

▷ Press on mid-line of the sacrum to test if movement of the sacroiliac joints is painful.

▷ Femoral stretch test: Flex the knee. If this does not trigger any pain, extend the leg at the hip. Pain suggests irritation of the second, third or fourth lumbar root of that side.

Ask the patient to lie supine.

▷ Straight leg raise: pain in the thigh, buttock and back suggests sciatica.

▷ The pain can also be elicited by concomitant dorsiflexion of the ankle (Bragard's test).

▷ Check out Lasegue's test if you're after a gold medal.

After the examination

Ask to perform neurological and vascular examinations.

Thank the patient.

Help the patient to put his clothes back on.

Offer a differential diagnosis.

Most common conditions likely to come up in an *Examine the spine* OSCE:

▷ Ankylosing spondylitis.

▷ Muscular back pain.

▷ Osteoarthritis.

▷ Scoliosis.

▷ Prolapsed disc.

73. Examine the hip

Before starting

Introduce yourself to the patient.

Explain the examination and ask for his consent to carry it out.

Ask him to undress to his undergarments.

Ensure that he is comfortable.

The examination

The patient is standing.

LOOK

- General inspection: posture, symmetry of legs and pelvis.
- Gait. Observe from front and back.
- Trendelenberg's test: Ask the patient to stand on each leg in turn, lifting the other one off the ground and bending it at the knee. The test is positive if the pelvis drops on the unsupported side.

Ask the patient to lie supine.

- Skin: colour, sinuses, scars.
- Position: limb shortening, limb rotation, abduction or adduction deformity, flexion deformity.
- Limb length:
  - To measure *true leg length*, position the pelvis so that the iliac crests lie in the same horizontal plane, at right angles to the trunk (if this is not possible there is a fixed abduction or adduction deformity) and then measure the distance from the anterior superior iliac spine to the medial malleolus. True limb shortening suggests pathology of the hip joint.
  - To measure *apparent leg length*, measure the distance from the xiphisternum to the medial malleolus.
- Circumference of quadriceps muscles at a fixed point.

FEEL

- Skin: temperature, effusions (difficult to feel).
- Bones and joints: bony landmarks of the hip joint, inguinal ligament.

MOVE

Look for limitation of the normal range of movement, and ask the patient to report any pain.

- Flexion:
  - Flex both hips.
  - Hold one hip flexed and straighten the other leg, keeping one hand in the small of the back.

If the leg cannot be straightened, there is a fixed flexion deformity (Thomas' test).

- ▷ Repeat for the other leg.
- ▷ Abduction and adduction:
  - ▷ Drop one leg over the edge of the couch to fix the pelvis.
  - ▷ Place one hand on the anterior superior iliac spine to fix the pelvis.
  - ▷ Carry the other leg through abduction and adduction.
  - ▷ Repeat for the other leg.
- ▷ Rotation:
  - ▷ Flex the hip and knee.
  - ▷ Hold the knee in the left hand and the ankle in the right hand.
  - ▷ Using your right hand, rotate the hip internally and externally.
  - ▷ Repeat for the other leg.

Ask the patient to lie prone.

- ▷ Look for scars, etc.
- ▷ Feel for tenderness.
- ▷ Extend each hip in turn.

After examining the hip

Ask to examine the vascular and neurological systems of the lower limbs.

Thank the patient.

Offer to help the patient put his clothes back on.

Offer a differential diagnosis.

 Most common conditions likely to come up in an *Examine the hip* OSCE:

- ▷ Osteoarthritis: hip in flexion, external rotation, and adduction, apparent limb shortening, pain, limp, limited range of movement, Heberden's nodes on distal interphalangeal joints.
- ▷ Hip replacement.
- ▷ Hip arthrodesis.
- ▷ Slipped upper femoral epiphysis.

74. Examine the knee

Before starting

Introduce yourself to the patient.

Explain the examination and ask for his consent to carry it out.

Ask him to remove his trousers.

Ensure that he is comfortable.

The examination

Patient is standing.

LOOK

- Gait: Observe from front and back looking for instability, limp and limited range of movement.
- Position: Neutral, varus, valgus, fixed flexion, hyperextension (recurvatum).
- Squat test (avoid in elderly patients).

Lie patient supine.

- Skin: Colour, sinuses, scars (including arthroscopic scars).
- Shape: Alignment, effusion, patellar alignment.
- Position: Fixed flexion.

Measure quadriceps circumference at a fixed point.

FEEL

- Skin: Temperature.
- Effusions: Patellar tap test and bulge sign.
- Joint line at 90 degrees of flexion.
- Synovial thickening.
- Surrounding structures: ligaments, tibial tuberosity, femoral condyles.
- Patella: Note size and height and carry out patellar apprehension test.

MOVE

- Active:
  - Flexion.
  - Extension.
  - Straight leg raise.
- Passive:
  - Flexion (to 140 degrees), feeling for crepitus and clicks.
  - Extension (to 0 degrees to −10 degrees).

Special tests

Collateral ligament tears

Apply varus and valgus stresses at 0 degrees and 20 degrees of flexion.

Cruciate ligament tears

- Posterior sag test: Flex knee to 90 degrees and look for a sag across the knee. The presence of a sag indicates a posterior cruciate ligament tear.
- Anterior and posterior drawer tests: flex knee to 90 degrees, sit on foot (ask the patient first!), and pull tibia back and forth.
- Lachman's test: Flex knee to 20 degrees and, holding the thigh in one hand and proximal tibia in the other, attempt to make the joint surfaces slide on one another.

Meniscal tears

- McMurray's test.
- Apley's grinding test (not usually performed).

Popliteal fossa

- Lie patient prone.
- Inspect the popliteal fossa.
- Palpate the popliteal fossa (Baker's cyst).

After the examination

Ask to examine the vascular and neurological systems of the lower limb.

Thank the patient.

Offer to help the patient put his clothes back on.

Offer a differential diagnosis.

! The age and sex of the patient have a strong bearing on the differential diagnosis.

> **Most common conditions likely to come up in an *Examine the knee* OSCE:**
>
> - Osteoarthritis.
> - Baker's (popliteal) cyst.
> - Prepatellar and infrapatellar bursitis.
> - Chondromalacia patellae.
> - Recurrent subluxation of the patella.
> - Tibial apophysitis (Osgood–Schlätter's disease).
> - Collateral ligament tears.
> - Cruciate ligament tears.
> - Meniscal tears.

75. Examine the ankle and foot

Before starting

Introduce yourself to the patient.

Explain the examination and ask for his consent to carry it out.

Ask him to remove his shoes and socks and to expose his entire leg.

Ensure that he is comfortable.

The examination

The patient is standing.

LOOK

- General inspection: posture, symmetry and any obvious deformities.
- Gait. Observe from front and back. Ask patient to stand on tiptoes and then on his heels.

Ask patient to lie on the couch.

- Skin: colour, sinuses, scars, corns, calluses.
- Shape: alignment, *pes planus*, *pes cavus*, deformities of the toes (*hallux valgus*, claw, mallet, and hammer toe).
- Position: varus or valgus hindfoot deformity.

FEEL

- Skin: temperature, abnormal thickening on soles of feet.
- Pulses.
- Bones and joints: palpate the forefoot and hindfoot and, looking at the patient's face, localise any tenderness.

MOVE

Look for restriction of the normal range of movement. Ask the patient to report any pain.

Ankle joint

- Hold the heel in the left hand and the forefoot in the right hand.
- Plantarflex the foot (normal range 40 degrees).
- Dorsiflex the foot (normal range 25 degrees).
- Compare range of movement to that in the other foot.

Subtalar joint

- Hold the heel in the left hand and the forefoot in the right hand, as above, with the ankle fixed at 90 degrees.
- Invert the foot (normal range 30 degrees).
- Evert the foot (normal range 30 degrees).
- Compare range of movement to that in the other foot.

Mid-tarsal joint

○ Hold the heel in the left hand and the forefoot in the right hand.

○ Flex, extend, invert and evert the forefoot.

Toes

○ Flex and extend each toe in turn. If there is any tenderness, try to localise it to a particular joint.

Muscle function

○ Test muscle function at each of the foot's joints.

○ Specifically test extensor hallucis longus.

Ask the patient to lie prone.

○ Look for any scars and for wasting of the calves.

○ Palpate the calf muscle and the Achilles' tendon (*tendo calcaneus*).

○ Squeeze the calf – if the foot plantarflexes, the Achilles' tendon is intact (Simmond's test).

After the examination

Ask to examine the vascular and neurological systems of the lower limb.

Thank the patient.

Offer to help the patient put his socks and shoes back on.

Offer a differential diagnosis.

	Most common conditions likely to come up in an *Examine the ankle and foot* OSCE:	
	○ Osteoarthritis.	○ Deformities of the foot.
	○ Rheumatoid arthritis.	○ Plantar fasciitis.
	○ Ankle injuries.	

76. Perform adult Basic Life Support

Specifications: A mannequin in lieu of a patient.

Ensure safe approach.

Shake and shout, "Are you all right?"

If there is no response, shout for help.

Airway

- Turn the patient on his back and open his airway by the head-tilt, chin-lift method. If cervical spine injury is a possibility, open his airway by the jaw-thrust method.
- Remove any visible obstruction from the mouth.

Breathing

- Holding the patient's airway open, put your ear to his mouth. *Listen*, *feel* and *look* for breathing for 10 seconds.

  → If he is breathing normally, place him in the recovery position and find help. Then reassess his breathing.

- If he is not breathing normally, immediately telephone for help. Note: If the patient is more likely to be unconscious because of a breathing problem than because of a heart problem (as in asphyxia, trauma or alcohol abuse), you should perform resuscitation for about one minute before finding help.
- Once you have called for help, give two effective rescue breaths, ensuring that the chest rises and falls. Don't forget to maintain the mouth open by head-tilt chin-lift and to pinch the nose closed. If after five attempts, despite having re-checked the mouth and having corrected your head-tilt, chin-lift technique, you still do not succeed in delivering two effective rescue breaths, move on.

Circulation

- Feel for the carotid pulse for 10 seconds. Never feel for both carotid pulses simultaneously.

  → If there are signs of circulation, continue rescue breathing and re-check for circulation every minute.

- If there are no signs of circulation, or you are unsure, begin external cardiac massage. Place the heels of your interlocked hands above the xiphoid and depress the chest by 4–5 cm. Aim for a compression rate of 100 per minute, delivering two rescue breaths for every 15 compressions.
- Stop and re-check circulation only if the patient makes a movement or takes a spontaneous breath. If not, continue until help arrives, or until exhaustion.

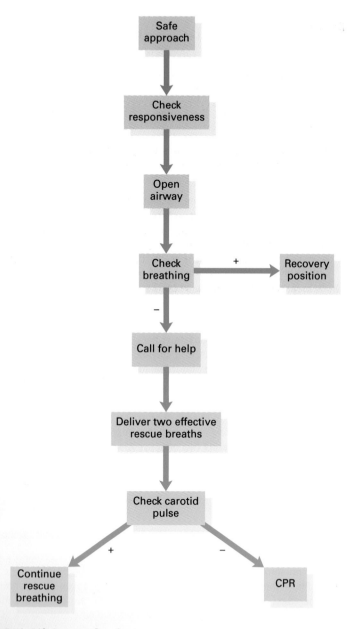

Figure 10. Basic Life Support flowchart

Choking

○ If the patient is conscious and breathing, encourage him to cough.

○ If the patient cannot breathe or is exhausted or cyanosed, remove any debris from the mouth and give up to five back blows.

○ If after five back blows the foreign body is not dislodged, give up to five abdominal thrusts.

○ If after five abdominal thrusts the foreign body is still not dislodged, check the mouth and continue the sequence of back blows and abdominal thrusts.

○ If, at any point, the patient becomes unconscious, begin Basic Life Support. If after five attempts effective breaths still cannot be delivered, do not check the pulse but start chest compressions immediately in an attempt to dislodge the foreign body. Check the mouth for any obstruction and attempt rescue breaths every 15 compressions. If you succeed in delivering an effective breath, check the pulse and continue chest compressions only if no pulse can be found.

77. Perform Advanced Life Support

Specifications: A mannequin in lieu of a patient.

The patient has arrested.

○ Attach the defibrillator or monitor and assess the rhythm: ventricular fibrillation and pulseless ventricular tachycardia are shockable rhythms.

○ Check the carotid pulse.

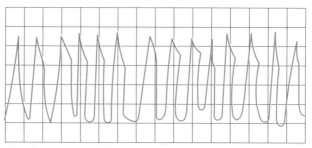

Ventricular tachycardia

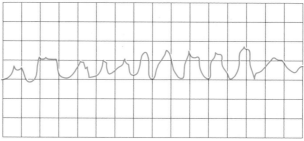

Ventricular fibrillation

Figure 11. ECG traces of ventricular fibrillation and of ventricular tachycardia

If this is a case of ventricular fibrillation or pulseless ventricular tachycardia, defibrillate.

Get ready

○ Position an electrode pad just inferior to the right clavicle and another just outside the cardiac apex.

○ Set the defibrillator to 200J.

○ Carry the paddles to the chest, placing the right paddle on the right pad and the left paddle on the left pad.

First attempt at defibrillation

- Charge the paddles to 200J.
- Shout "All clear" and "Oxygen away", and perform a visual check of the area.
- Defibrillate at 200J.
- Maintain the paddles on the patient's chest and assess the rhythm. (If the rhythm is ventricular tachycardia or if it changes to a rhythm that can sustain an output, also check the pulse.)

Second attempt at defibrillation

- Recharge the defibrillator.
- Shout "All clear" and perform a visual check of the area.
- Defibrillate at 200J.
- Maintain the paddles on the patient's chest and assess the rhythm. (If the rhythm is ventricular tachycardia or if it changes to a rhythm that can sustain an output, also check the pulse.)

Third attempt at defibrillation

- Ask an assistant to set the defibrillator to 360J, or return one paddle to the defibrillator and use your free hand to set the defibrillator to 360J.
- Recharge the defibrillator.
- Shout "All clear" and perform a visual check of the area.
- Defibrillate at 360J.
- Return the paddles to the defibrillator and assess the rhythm. (If the rhythm is ventricular tachycardia or if it changes to a rhythm that can sustain an output, check the pulse.)

! **Try to administer the three shocks in less than one minute.**

If the first cycle of defibrillation is unsuccessful

- Perform cardiopulmonary resuscitation for one minute (see Chapter 76, *Perform adult Basic Life Support*).
- During that time:
  - Get the patient intubated (using either an endotracheal tube or a laryngeal mask) and ventilated on 100% oxygen. Once the patient is intubated, ventilation and chest compressions can be carried out simultaneously.
  - Place a peripheral cannula and administer 1 mg of adrenaline, equivalent to 10 ml of a 1 in 10000 solution.
  - So long as this does not delay the delivery of the fourth shock, administer 300 mg of amiodarone.
  - Check the positions of the electrode pads and of the paddles.

○ If at the end of the minute the patient is still in ventricular fibrillation or pulseless ventricular tachycardia, deliver three further shocks at 360J and start one minute of cardiopulmonary resuscitation. Continue this process, remembering to administer 1 mg of adrenaline every three minutes and to check the pulse regularly.

If the arrhythmia is persistent, try changing the position of the paddles to anterior–posterior, or using another defibrillator. Continue resuscitation for as long as the patient is in ventricular fibrillation or pulseless ventricular tachycardia.

Consider the reversible causes of a cardiac arrest

Hypoxia.

Hypovolaemia.

Hyperkalaemia, hypocalcaemia or acidaemia.

Hypothermia.

Tension pneumothorax.

Tamponade.

Toxic substances.

Thromboembolism.

Non-shockable rhythms

ASYSTOLE

Ensure that the patient is truly in asystole (check the leads and the gain); if in doubt treat as for ventricular fibrillation. Perform Basic Life Support for 3 minutes. During that time, intubate, place a cannula, and deliver 1 mg of adrenaline and 3 mg of atropine. After 3 minutes, assess the rhythm and check the pulse. If the patient remains in asystole, continue Basic Life Support, delivering 1 mg of adrenaline every 3 minutes. Assess the rhythm and check the pulse every 3 minutes. Identify and treat any underlying causes.

ELECTROMECHANICAL DISSOCIATION (PULSELESS ELECTRICAL ACTIVITY)

Perform Basic Life Support for 3 minutes. During that time, intubate, place a cannula and deliver 1 mg of adrenaline and, if the heart rate is less than 60 beats per minute, 3 mg of atropine. After 3 minutes, assess the rhythm and check the pulse. If the patient remains in electromechanical dissociation, continue Basic Life Support, delivering 1 mg of adrenaline every 3 minutes. Assess the rhythm and check the pulse every three minutes. Identify and treat any underlying causes.

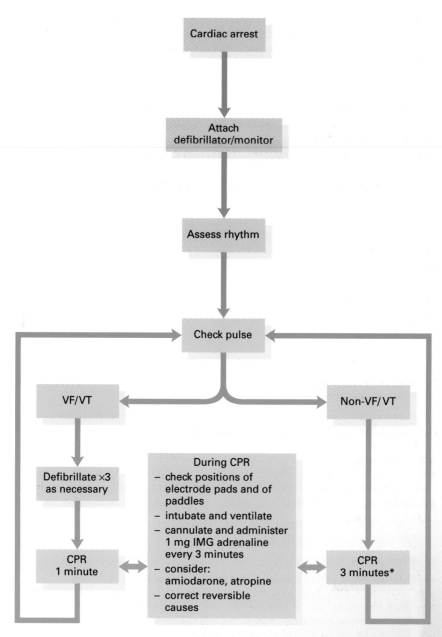

*1 minute if immediately after defibrillation

Figure 12. Advanced Life Support flow chart

78. The primary and secondary surveys

The quick look

- Look at the patient.
- Introduce yourself to the patient. Is the patient responsive?
- If the patient is unconscious, try to elicit a response by shouting out his name.

Airway and cervical spine

- Immobilise the cervical spine in a stiff collar. Place sandbags on either side of the head and tape them across the forehead.
- Assess the airway.
- If appropriate, clear and secure the airway. A jaw thrust is often all that is required.

Breathing

- Assess breathing: look, listen and feel.
- Note the rate and depth of respiration.
- Look for any chest injuries.
- Palpate for tracheal shift. Palpate, percuss and auscultate the chest. Exclude flail segments, pneumothorax and haemothorax.
- Attach a pulse oximeter.
- If appropriate, ventilate using a bag, mask and oropharyngeal airway or endotracheal tube.

Circulation

- Control any visible haemorrhage by direct pressure.
- Assess the pulse.
- Assess skin colour, capillary refill time, JVP, heart sounds and blood pressure. Exclude cardiac tamponade.
- Attach an ECG monitor.
- Place two large-calibre cannulas into large peripheral veins.
- Take a sample of blood for group and cross-match.
- Start fluid replacement.

Disability

Assess neurological function on the AVPU scale.

A   Alert.

V   Voice elicits a response.

P   Pain elicits a response.

U   Unresponsive.

Assess the pupils for size and reactivity.

Check that all extremities can be moved.

Exposure

Remove all the patient's clothing and inspect both his front and back. Log-roll him so that his spine is immobilised.

Secondary survey

Once the patient is stable

- ▷ Take a short history:
    - ▷ **A**llergies
    - ▷ **M**edications and tetanus immunity
    - ▷ **P**revious medical history
    - ▷ **L**ast meal
    - ▷ **E**vents leading to the injury
- ▷ Carry out a head-to-toe physical examination.
- ▷ Monitor ECG, BP, oxygen saturation and core temperature.
- ▷ Insert a urinary catheter and a naso-gastric tube.
- ▷ Order investigations: full blood count, urea and electrolytes, liver function tests, amylase, glucose, coagulation profile, arterial blood gases, toxicology screen and X-rays of the lateral cervical spine, chest and pelvis.

79. Ventilate with a bag-valve mask

Assess the patient

Check that the airway is patent and remove any visible obstruction from the mouth.

Ensure that the patient is not breathing. Holding the airway open, put your ear to the mouth and *listen*, *feel* and *look* for breathing for 10 seconds.

Check the carotid pulse. Is the patient in cardiac arrest? (See *Perform Advanced Life Support*, Chapter 77).

Request help.

The procedure

- Do a head tilt–chin lift. If C-spine injury has not been excluded, do a jaw thrust.
- Identify the need for an airway. If a Guedel airway is required, size it by measuring the distance from the incisors to the angle of the jaw. If there is a gag reflex, consider inserting a naso-pharyngeal tube instead.
- Choose an appropriately sized mask.
- Attach the bag-valve mask to an oxygen supply. Adjust the flow rate to 15L per minute.
- Hold the mask over the face with your dominant hand. Place your thumb over the nose and support the jaw with the middle or ring fingers. Ensure a tight seal.
- Do a head tilt–chin lift.
- Use your free hand to compress the bag.
- Look for a rise in the chest.

! If you have help, hold the mask in both hands and get the other person to squeeze the bag.

- Ventilate at a rate of 12 compressions per minute until the patient starts breathing or until the patient can be intubated and put on a ventilator.

80. Insert a laryngeal mask airway

Specifications: A mannequin in lieu of a patient.

⟶ **Laryngeal mask sizes:**

Size 1	Infant
Size 2	Child
Size 3	Small adult
Size 4	Large adult

Equipment

- Laryngeal mask.
- Lubricant.
- Air-filled syringe.
- Bandage.

Before inserting the laryngeal mask

Assemble equipment.

Lubricate mask.

Ensure adequate depth of analgesia (cough reflex should be suppressed).

Ensure that the patient has been pre-oxygenated, or pre-oxygenate him by bag ventilation.

Perform a head tilt so that the mouth is fully open.

Check state of the teeth.

Inserting the laryngeal mask

- Insert the tip of the mask into the mouth, ensuring that the aperture is facing the tongue.
- Press the tip of the mask against the hard palate as you introduce it into the pharynx.
- Use your index finger to guide the tube into the pharynx until resistance is felt.
- Check that the black line on the tube faces the upper lip.

   → If you do not succeed in inserting the laryngeal mask, you must pre-oxygenate the patient a second time before you try again.

After inserting the laryngeal mask

Inflate the cuff, ensuring that you do not over-inflate it. A size 3 mask needs 25 ml of air; a size 4 requires 35 ml.

Secure the cuff in place by means of a length of bandage.

Attach the breathing system and check that the patient is being satisfactorily ventilated.

81. Suture a wound

Specifications: A pad of "skin" in lieu of a patient.

! **This OSCE station most likely only requires you to talk through the procedure, or parts of the procedure, and then to demonstrate your suturing skills.**

Before starting

Introduce yourself to the patient.

Explain the procedure and ask for his consent to carry it out.

Examine the wound. Debris and dirt require cleaning and debridement.

Ask for an X-ray to exclude a foreign body, if appropriate.

Assess distal motor and sensory function.

Position the patient appropriately and ensure that he is comfortable.

Equipment

Gather:

- A pair of sterile gloves.
- A suture pack.
- A suture of appropriate type and size.
- A syringe, two green needles, and a vial of local anaesthetic.
- Antiseptic solution.
- A sharps bin.

The procedure

- Wash your hands.
- Open the sterile pack, thus creating a sterile field.
- Pour antiseptic solution into the receptacle.
- Open the sterile gloves, the suture, the syringe and both needles onto the sterile field.
- Wash your hands using sterile technique.
- Don the sterile gloves.
- Attach a needle to the syringe.
- Ask an assistant to open the vial of local anaesthetic and draw 5 ml of local anaesthetic.
- Discard the needle in the sharps bin and attach the second needle to the syringe.
- Clean the skin (use forceps) and drape the field.

- Inject the local anaesthetic. Make sure to pull back on the plunger before injecting. Discard the needle in the sharps bin.
- Give the anaesthetic 5–10 minutes to work.
- Apply sutures 5–10 mm apart. Use toothed forceps to hold the needle and forceps to pick up the skin margins. Knot the sutures around the toothed forceps.

After the procedure

Dress the wound.

Assess the need for a tetanus injection.

Give appropriate instructions for wound care and indicate the date sutures are to be removed (about 7 days for most wounds).

Ask if the patient has any questions or concerns.

Thank the patient.

82. Prescribe a drug

Before prescribing a drug

Find out if the patient has any allergies and document them.

Find out if he has liver or kidney impairment/failure.

Find out if he is on any other drugs, and consider possible interactions.

Explain to the patient the reason for the drug, its likely effects and its common or dangerous side-effects.

Prescribing a drug

◯ Write legibly and in black ink.

◯ Avoid all abbreviations others than those that are in common usage (see *Common Latin abbreviations used in drug prescriptions* box).

◯ Use generic names (unless a particular drug preparation is required).

Include:

◯ The date.

◯ The full name, address and date of birth of the patient.

◯ The age of the patient if he is a child under the age of 12 (prescription-only medicines only).

◯ The generic name and formulation of the drug.

◯ The dose and frequency. Use the most appropriate units, e.g., 500 mg and not 0.5 g.

◯ The minimum dose interval (for "as required" drugs only).

◯ The quantity to be supplied.

◯ The signature of a registered medical practitioner.

! Any alterations or mistakes should be initialled.

Prescribing a controlled drug

In your own handwriting, include the:

◯ Date.

◯ Name, address and date of birth of the patient.

◯ Generic name of the drug.

◯ Formulation and strength of the preparation.

◯ Total amount of the preparation, or the number of dose units in both words *and* numbers.

◯ Required dose of the drug, frequency and number of days it is to be taken.

◯ Your signature and address.

Common Latin abbreviations used in drug prescriptions:

Abbreviation	Latin	English
o.d.	omni die	once a day
b.d.	bis in die	twice a day
t.d.s	ter die sumendus	three times a day
q.d.s.	quater die sumendus	four times a day
q.q.h.	quarta quaque horae	every four hours
a.c.	ante cibum	before food
p.c.	post cibum	after food
o.m.	omni mane	in the morning
o.n.	omni nocte	at night
p.r.n.	pro re nata	as required
Stat.	statim	immediately

If you are unsure about a drug, check the British National Formulary.

After prescribing a drug

Give the patient instructions for administration of the drug.

Ask the patient if he has any questions or concerns.

83. Confirm death

Golden lads and girls all must,
As chimney-sweepers, come to dust.

Cymbeline: Act II, Scene 2

Shakespeare

Specifications: A mannequin in lieu of a corpse(!)

- ▷ Take a history from a nurse (or indicate that you would do so) and consider the need for resuscitation.
- ▷ Ask for the patient's notes.
- ▷ Confirm the patient's identity: check his name tag.
- ▷ Observe the patient's general appearance and note the absence of respiratory movements.
- ▷ Ascertain that the patient does not rouse to verbal or tactile stimuli, such as pressure on a nail-bed.
- ▷ Confirm that the pupils are fixed and dilated.
- ▷ Feel for the carotid pulses *on both sides*.
- ▷ Feel for the radial pulses.
- ▷ Feel for the femoral pulses.
- ▷ Auscultate over the precordium. Indicate that you would listen for one minute. Does the patient have a pacemaker?
- ▷ Auscultate over the lungs. Indicate that you would listen for 3 minutes.

! **If any of your findings are non-corroboratory, you must consider the need for resuscitation.**

- ▷ Make an entry in the patient's notes. Remember to include the time and the date, and to sign the entry.
- ▷ Indicate that you would:
    - ▷ Consider the need for a post-mortem (see Chapter 84, *Complete a death certificate*).
    - ▷ Complete a death certificate (see Chapter 84).
    - ▷ Inform the patient's GP and next of kin of the patient's death.

84. Complete a death certificate

Legally, you can only fill in the death certificate if you have seen the patient in his last 14 days. Once the certificate is completed, it should be taken to the Registrar of Births and Deaths, usually by the patient's next of kin.

Before starting

You must understand the patient's history and the circumstances surrounding his death. You should have seen the patient's body to confirm his death (or had the patient's body seen by a medically qualified colleague), noted if he had a pacemaker or radioactive implant, phoned his GP and considered the need for a post-mortem examination (see *Some reasons for referral to a coroner* box).

Filling in the death certificate

In black ink, and as clearly and precisely as possible:

- Fill in the patient's:
  - Name.
  - Date of death.
  - Age.
  - Place of death.
- Fill in the date on which you last saw the patient alive.
- Circle one of the following statements:
  1. The certified cause of death takes account of information obtained from post-mortem.
  2. Information from post-mortem may be available later.
  3. Post-mortem not being held.
  4. I have reported this death to the Coroner for further action.
- Circle one of the following statements:
  a) Seen after death by me.
  b) Seen after death by another medical practitioner but not by me.
  c) Not seen after death by a medical practitioner.
- Fill in the cause of death: the disease that lead directly to the patient's death is entered in section I (a). The diseases that lead to the disease entered in section I (a) are entered in sections I (b) and I (c).
- Fill in other significant diseases contributing to the death but not related to the disease having caused it in section II.
- Tick the relevant box if the death is related to employment.

▷ Sign the death certificate, fill in the date of issue and print your name and medical qualification(s).

▷ Fill in the name of the consultant responsible for the overall care of the patient.

▷ Fill in the Counterfoil: record the patient's details and circumstances of death.

▷ Fill in the Note to Informant, and give it to the next of kin.

Some reasons for referral to a coroner:

▷ The cause of death is uncertain.

▷ The cause of death is due to industrial disease.

▷ The cause of death is accidental.

▷ The cause of death is violent.

▷ The cause of death is suspicious.

▷ The death is related to surgery or anaesthesia.

▷ A doctor has not attended in the 14 days prior to the patient's death.

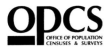

**OFFICE OF POPULATION
CENSUSES & SURVEYS**

Medical Statistics Division

St Catherine's House
10 Kingsway
London WC2B 6JP

Telephone: 071-242 0262
Extension:
GTN: 3042

Fax: 071-404 1186

May 1990

Dear Doctor,

COMPLETION OF MEDICAL CERTIFICATES OF CAUSE OF DEATH

As you are aware the medical certificates of cause of death which you complete, for transmission to the Registrar of Births and Deaths serve both legal and statistical purposes. Our general experience in the handling of death certificates shows that most certifying doctors are punctilious and precise in completing them. However, we have identified certain aspects of certificate completion where ambiguities in our advice may have contributed to our receiving a number of less than satisfactory certificates. We thus wish to draw the attention of doctors to these aspects, which cover the recording of **modes of dying**, the recording of **diseases which might have been due to previous employment**, and the use of **abbreviations.** In this letter reference is made from time to time to the existing notes (which are provided with blank medical certificates of cause of death).

MODES OF DYING

Under current regulations Registrars of Births and Deaths are required to report to the Coroner any death the cause of which appears to be unknown, and a death where the Medical Certificate of Cause of Death shows **only** the mode of dying is usually deemed to fall within this requirement.

Present guidance to certifiers (on page iii of the notes) regarding the nature and status of conditions which may be considered as modes of dying states:-

> ".... there is no need to record the mode of dying (such as heart failure or asphyxia). Addition of a statement of the mode of dying does not assist in deriving mortality statistics, where the underlying cause of death is explicitly stated (eg Cardiac Arrest following Myocardial Infarct.). Even more important is the need to avoid completing a certificate with the mode of dying as the only entry; this should be the subject of further enquiry if the disease process involved is genuinely not known."

The guidance to advisable practice summarised as **"..avoid completing a certificate with the mode of dying as the only entry,"** is generally taken in the context of the statistical, rather than the legal consequences of non-adherence; you are reminded that, for the reasons given above, non-compliance may well result in the referral of the case to the Coroner.

Statements which imply a mode of dying rather than a cause of death

I would like you to know that a more comprehensive list of 'unacceptable' statements has been constructed, and is reproduced here for your information:

Asphyxia	Asthenia
Brain failure	Cachexia
Cardiac arrest	Cardiac failure (not further qualified)
Coma	Debility (General)
Exhaustion	Heart failure (not further qualified)
Hepatic failure	Hepatorenal failure
Kidney failure	Liver failure
Liver and kidney failure	Renal failure
Respiratory arrest	Shock
Syncope	Uraemia
Vagal inhibition	Vasovagal attack

The primary purpose of the provision of this detailed list is to assist you in completion of Medical Certificates of Cause of Death. However, this list is also being supplied to all Registrars of Births and Deaths, with instructions that when any of these statements is **used alone on a Medical Certificate** it should be interpreted by them as a mode of dying rather than as a definitive cause of death, and normally referred to the Coroner. It should be further noted that, except where specified, the simple qualification of the terms in this list by such words as 'acute' or 'chronic' **is not sufficient to make them acceptable.**

Whenever certifiers have insufficient knowledge regarding the cause of death over and above an awareness of the mode of dying, it is, of course, a requirement for such deaths to be reported to Coroners. However this course of action should not normally be necessary in a situation in which the certifying doctor has knowledge of a relevant natural underlying cause, but merely fails to record it. I would thus like to remind you of your statutory responsibilities regarding the provision of a cause of death (as specified on page i of the notes), and which require you in all cases to state it 'to the best of your knowledge and belief'.

DEATHS THAT MIGHT BE DUE TO PREVIOUS EMPLOYMENT

I should further like to remind you of your obligations, (detailed on page ii of the notes) regarding the completion of medical certificates, and the reporting to Coroners of deaths which might be due to or contributed by the employment followed at some time by the deceased. Some diseases, such as tuberculosis, which in some circumstances may be employment-related are often known not to be so in the case of a particular deceased person. In these instances qualification on the death certificate by a form of words such as 'non-industrial' can preclude subsequent enquiries by the Registrar of Births and Deaths.

ABBREVIATIONS

All doctors will be aware of the misunderstandings that can arise by the recording of even the most commonly used abbreviations. It is thus important that certifiers should refrain from this practice when completing certificates of cause of Death. Failure to do so may also generate further enquiries by Registrars of Births and Deaths.

NEED FOR ACTION

If it is necessary for Registrars of Births and Deaths to take further action, or to make further enqiries, this can can cause anxieties to relatives of deceased persons, and delay arrangements that they may have made. Thus I would be grateful for your co-operation in noting the matters identified in this letter and taking such action as is required.

I have arranged for this letter to be distributed to General Practitioners through Family Practitioner Committees; and to Hospital Consultants through Regional Medical Officers. In due course it is also expected that the printed instructions incorporated in the blank books of certificates will be updated, but in the meantime Registrars of Births and Deaths will also include a copy of this letter when a futher supply of certificates is ordered.

It would be very helpful if you could assist us further by bringing it to the attention of any of your colleagues who would not have received it directly through these channels.

Yours sincerely

Dr J S A Ashley   MB FFCM
Deputy Chief Medical Statistician

COUNTERFOIL

For use of Medical Practitioner, who should complete in all cases.

Name of
deceased

Date of death

Age

Place of death

Last seen alive }
by me

Post-mortem/*   1   2   3   4
Coroner

Whether seen   a   b   c
after death*

Cause of death:—

I

  (a)

  (b)

  (c)

II

Employment?   ☐   *Please tick where applicable*

B. Further information offered?

Signature

Date

Ring appropriate digit(s) and letter.

Register to enter
No. of Death Entry

☐

BIRTHS AND DEATHS REGISTRATION ACT 1953

(Form prescribed by the Registration of Births and Death Registration Regulations (1987))

MEDICAL CERTIFICATE OF CAUSE OF DEATH

For use only by a Registered Medical Practitioner WHO HAS BEEN IN ATTENDANCE during the deceased's last illness, and to be delivered by him forthwith to the Registrar of Births and Deaths.

Name of deceased

Date of death as stated to me .... day of ....

Place of death .... day of ....

Last seen alive by me .... Age as stated to me ....

1   The certified cause of death takes account of information   a   Seen after death by me.
    obtained from post-mortem.

2   Information from post-mortem may be available later.   b   Seen after death by another medical practitioner but not by me.

3   Post-mortem not being held.   *Please ring appropriate digit(s) and letter*

4   I have reported this death to the Coroner for further action.   c   Not seen after death by a medical practitioner.
    [See overleaf]

CAUSE OF DEATH

The condition thought to be the 'Underlying Cause of Death' should appear in the lowest completed line of Part I.

                      These particulars not to be entered in death register

                      Approximate interval between onset and death

I (a)   Disease or condition directly leading to death†

  (b)   Other disease or condition, if any, leading to I(a)

  (c)   Other disease or condition, if any, leading to I(b)

II   Other significant conditions CONTRIBUTING TO THE DEATH but not related to the disease or condition causing it.

SAMPLE

The death might have been due to or contributed to by the employment followed at some time by the deceased.   ☐   *Please tick where applicable*

†*This does not mean the mode of dying, such as heart failure, asphyxia, asthenia, etc: it means the disease, injury, or complication which caused death.*

I hereby certify that I was in medical attendance during the above named deceased's last illness, and that the particulars and cause of death above written are true to the best of my knowledge and belief.

Signature .... Qualifications as registered by General Medical Council }

Residence .... Date ....

For deaths in hospital: Please give the name of the consultant responsible for the above-named as a patient.

(Form prescribed by the Registration of Births and Deaths Regulations 1987)

NOTICE TO INFORMANT

I hereby give notice that I have this day signed a medical certificate of cause of death of

....

Signature ....

Date ....

This notice is to be delivered by the informant to the registrar of births and deaths for the sub-district in which the death occurred.

The certifying medical practitioner must give this notice to the person who is qualified and liable to act as informant for the registration of death (see list overleaf). Where the informant intends giving information for the registration outside of the area where the death occurred, this notice may be handed to the informant's agent.

DUTIES OF INFORMANT

Failure to deliver this notice to the registrar renders the informant liable to prosecution. The death cannot be registered until the medical certificate has reached the registrar.

When the death is registered the informant must be prepared to give to the registrar the following particulars relating to the deceased:

1. The date and place of death.
2. The full name and surname (and the maiden surname if the deceased was a woman who had married).
3. The date and place of birth.
4. The occupation (and if the deceased was a married woman or a widow the name and occupation of her husband).
5. The usual address.
6. Whether the deceased was in receipt of a pension or allowance from public funds.
7. If the deceased was married, the date of birth of the surviving widow or widower.

THE DECEASED'S MEDICAL CARD SHOULD BE DELIVERED TO THE REGISTRAR

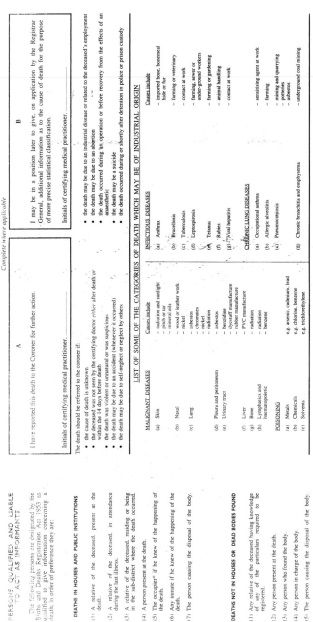

Figure 13. Death certificate

85. Explaining skills

These skills can be used to explain a common condition, to explain an investigation or to explain a procedure or treatment.

What to do

- Introduce yourself.
- Summarise the patient's presenting symptoms.
- Tell the patient what you are going to explain.
- Determine how much the patient already knows.
- Determine how much the patient would like to know.
- Deliver the information.
- Summarise and check understanding.
- Encourage and address questions.

How to do it

- Be empathic.
- Explore the patient's feelings.
- Give the most important information first.
- Be specific.
- Regularly check understanding.
- Pitch the explanation at the patient's level. Use simple language and short sentences. If using a medical or technical term, explain it in layman's terms.
- Use diagrams, if appropriate.
- Give a leaflet.
- Be honest. If you are unsure about something, say you will find out later and get back to the patient.

What not to do

- Hurry.
- Reassure too soon.
- Be patronising.
- Give too much information.
- Use medical jargon.
- Confabulate (make things up).

'Really, now you ask me,' said Alice, very much confused, 'I don't think—'
'Then you shouldn't talk,' said the Hatter.

Alice's Adventures in Wonderland: A Mad Tea-Party.

Lewis Carroll

86. Obtaining consent

The purpose of gaining consent

Consent is needed on every occasion a doctor wishes to initiate an investigation or treatment or any other intervention, except in emergencies or where the law dictates otherwise (such as where compulsory treatment is authorised by mental health legislation). Consent can be verbal or written. It is the quality and clarity of the information given that is of paramount consideration. Patients can also change their minds about a decision at any time, as long as they have the capacity to do so.

How long is consent valid?

Consent should be seen as a continuing process rather than a one-off decision. However, when there has been a significant period of time between the patient agreeing to a treatment option and its start, consent should be reaffirmed.

Refusal of treatment

Competent adult patients are entitled to refuse treatment even when doing so may result in permanent physical injury or death. For example, a Jehovah's Witness can refuse a blood transfusion even if he will die as a result.

Gaining consent (guidelines)

The type of information that should be provided to obtain consent includes:

- The reason for the procedure and its likely benefits.
- Details of the diagnosis, if any.
- Alternatives to the procedure, including the option not to investigate or not to treat.
- Explanation of the likely benefits and probabilities of success for each alternative.
- The nature and risk of side-effects for each alternative.
- The name of the doctor taking on overall responsibility for the procedure.
- A reminder that the patient can change his mind at any time.

Direct questions from the patient should be encouraged and replied to honestly.

Lastly, ensure that the information has been understood by the patient, and that the patient is competent to consent to treatment.

To demonstrate competence a patient should be able to:

- Understand what the procedure is and why it is being proposed.
- Understand its principal benefits, risks and alternatives.
- Understand in broad terms what the consequences of refusing it are.
- Retain the information for long enough to make an effective decision.
- Make a free decision.

87. Breaking bad news

What to do

- Introduce yourself.
- Look to comfort and privacy.
- Determine what the patient already knows.
- Determine what the patient would like to know.
- Warn the patient that bad news is coming.
- Break the bad news.
- Identify the patient's main concerns.
- Summarise and check understanding.
- Offer realistic hope.
- Arrange follow-up.
- Try to ensure there is someone with the patient when he leaves.

How to do it

- Be sensitive.
- Be empathic.
- Maintain eye contact.
- Give information in small chunks.
- Repeat and clarify.
- Regularly check understanding.
- Give the patient time to respond. Do not be afraid of silence and of tears.
- Explore the patient's emotions.
- Use physical contact.
- Be honest. If you are unsure about something, say you will find out later and get back to the patient.

What not to do

- Hurry.
- Give all the information in one go, or give too much information.
- Use euphemisms or medical jargon.
- Lie or be economical with the truth.
- Be blunt. Words are loaded pistols, as Jean-Paul Sartre once said.
- Prognosticate (*"she's got six months, maybe seven"*).

88. The angry patient

I was angry with my friend:
I told my wrath, my wrath did end.
I was angry with my foe:
I told it not, my wrath did grow.

William Blake.

The "angry patient" station can be rather unnerving, if only because medical students – and especially medical students in the earlier years of their training – have not heretofore confronted such patients.

The aim of the game is to diffuse the patient's anger, not to rationalise it or to placate it. You should therefore try to be as empathic as possible.

What to do

- Introduce yourself.
- Acknowledge the patient's anger.
- Try to find the reason for his anger, e.g., frustration, fear, guilt.
- Validate his feelings.
- Let him vent his anger, or any feelings that led to his anger, e.g., frustration, fear, guilt.
- Offer to do something or for him to do something.

How to do it

- Sit at the same level as the patient, not too close to him but not too far either.
- Make eye contact.
- Speak calmly and do not raise your voice.
- Avoid dismissive or threatening body language.
- Encourage the patient to speak. Ask open rather than closed questions, and use verbal and non-verbal cues to show that you are listening.
- Empathise as much as you can.

What not to do

- Glare at the patient.
- Confront him.
- Interrupt him.
- Patronise him.
- Get too close to or touch him.
- Block his exit route.
- Put the blame on others.
- Make unreasonable promises.

89. Talk to a patient about discharge

Setting the scene

- Introduce yourself to the patient.
- Summarise the situation to the patient.
- Explore the impact that the illness/hospitalisation has had on the patient.
- Explore the patient's current mood and dispositions.

Going home and after

- Explain that you are considering for the patient to go home.
- Elicit and address any concerns that the patient might have about going home.
- Reassure the patient that transport can be organised, if need be.
- Explore the patient's home situation and support system.
- Consider any extra help that can be offered to the patient, for example, social services, home help, *meals on wheels*, health visitor, district nurse, specialist nurses, palliative care team, dietician, occupational therapist, speech therapist, physiotherapist, psychologist, continence advisor, self-help group, day centre.
- Medication and compliance. Check that the patient doesn't have any concerns about taking his discharge medication.
- Risk factors. Suggest lifestyle changes that the patient can benefit from, such as stopping smoking, eating a balanced diet, taking regular exercise, etc.
- Offer the patient a follow-up appointment either at his GPs or in the Out-Patients' Department.

Before finishing

- Summarise what has been said.
- Check the patient's understanding of what has been said.
- Ask the patient if he has any further questions or concerns.
- Thank the patient.

90. Cross-cultural communication

You do not need to have a masters in anthropology from the School of Oriental and African Studies to score highly in this OSCE station. All you need to do is use some basic communication strategies, as detailed here. It is also important that you are seen to respect the patient's beliefs and/or values.

- Introduce yourself to the patient, and ensure that he is comfortable.
- Ask the patient's name, age and occupation.
- Determine the patient's reason for attending.
- Elicit the patient's:
  - Ideas.
  - Concerns.
  - Expectations.

(ICE)

- Establish:
  - The patient's cultural or religious group.
  - The implications that this has on his reason for attending.
  - The patient's individual beliefs and values.
- Check that you have understood the patient's problem.
- Explore possible solutions, and agree on a mutually satisfactory course of action.
- Summarise the consultation.
- Check the patient's understanding.
- Thank the patient.